300 Single Best Answers

for the
Final FRCR Part A

D1447651

300 Single Best Answers

for the
Final FRCR Part A

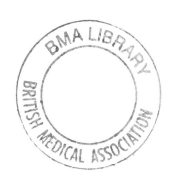

Chaitanya Gupta MRCS FRCR
Consultant Radiologist
Northern Lincoln & Goole Hospitals NHS Foundation Trust
UK

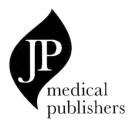

JP
medical
publishers

London • St Louis • Panama City • New Delhi

© 2010 JP Medical Ltd.
Published by JP Medical Ltd
83 Victoria Street, London, SW1H 0HW, UK
Tel: +44 (0)20 3170 8910
Fax: +44 (0)20 3008 6180
Email: info@jpmedpub.com
Web: www.jpmedpub.com

ISBN: 978-1-907816-02-4

British Library Cataloguing in Publication Data
A catalogue record for this book is available from the British Library

Library of Congress Cataloging in Publication Data
A catalog record for this book is available from the Library of Congress

JP Medical Ltd is a subsidiary of Jaypee Brothers Medical Publishers (P) Ltd, New Delhi, India with offices in Ahmedabad, Bengaluru, Chennai, Hyderabad, Kochi, Kolkata, Lucknow, Mumbai and Nagpur. Visit www.jaypeebrothers.com for more details.

Publisher:	Richard Furn
Development Editor:	Alison Whitehouse
Design:	Pete Wilder, Designers Collective Ltd

Typeset, printed and bound in India.

Preface

The Royal College of Radiologists has recently changed the pattern of the Final FRCR Part A examination from the multiple choice question (MCQ) format to single best answers (SBA). There have been a few examinations since the introduction of the new format and looking at some of the questions that have been asked, it is obvious that the questions have been written with daily radiology practice in mind.

The chapters in this book are organised in accordance with the six modules of the examination, with 50 questions in each module. In writing the questions I have tried to cover the common conditions that we come across in our day-to-day practice, although I have included unusual cases as well, which some examiners like to focus on in the area of their expertise.

Emphasis has been placed on cross-sectional imaging, including CT and MRI, with some mention of PET scanning as well. The recent literature has been scrutinised to be sure of reflecting current knowledge and imaging practice. Each answer is briefly discussed to explain why it is the single best answer.

Although the examination pattern has changed, the most important factor underpinning success is an understanding of the basic principles of imaging and disease processes so that the best answer will fall into place. I hope that this book will become a 'must-have' for all candidates sitting the examination, and wish readers the best of luck.

Chaitanya Gupta
July 2010

Acknowledgements

I am grateful for the support of my consultant radiology colleagues, who have provided advice and opinion on many cases.

In particular, I would like to express my gratitude to Dr Deepak Pai, Dr Ajay Dabra and Dr Sadashiv Kamath, who gave very useful ideas for some of the cases we discussed over lunch.

I would also like to thank my wife, Gunjan, for her patience as I spent many an hour on the computer.

Chaitanya Gupta

Contents

Chapter 1

Cardiothoracic and vascular system

QUESTIONS

1. A 70-year-old male presents to his GP with cough. The chest radiograph shows bilateral egg shell calcifications in the hilar regions.

    Which of the following is the least likely diagnosis?

    (a) Silicosis
    (b) Asbestosis
    (c) Coal workers pneumoconiosis
    (d) Sarcoidosis
    (e) Histoplasmosis

2. In a case of anaphylaxis, the proper dose of intramuscular adrenaline injection is?

    (a) 1 mL of 1:1000 adrenaline
    (b) 0.5 mL of 1:1000 adrenaline
    (c) 1 mL of 1:10,000 adrenaline
    (d) 1 mL of 1:10,000 adrenaline
    (e) 10 mL of 1:1000 adrenaline

3. A chest radiograph shows diffuse lung disease with fibrotic changes predominantly affecting the upper lobes.

    What is the most unlikely diagnosis?

    (a) Sarcoidosis
    (b) Cystic fibrosis
    (c) Allergic bronchopulmonary aspergillosis
    (d) Langerhans cell granulomatosis
    (e) Scleroderma

4. A 25-year-old man of African origin presents with dry cough. The chest radiograph shows bilateral lobulated hilar shadows. HRCT shows bilateral hilar and paratracheal lymphadenopathy with irregular and nodular septal thickening and traction bronchiectasis. Blood tests show elevated serum angiotensin-converting enzyme.

The most likely diagnosis is?

   (a) Lymphoma
   (b) Sarcoidosis
   (c) Malignant lymphangitis
   (d) Tuberculosis
   (e) Sjögren's syndrome

5. A 50-year-old man with recently diagnosed pancreatic cancer presents with acute onset of chest pain and dyspnoea. The chest radiograph is normal. A V/Q scan is performed. Perfusion images show multiple segmental filling defects and the ventilation images show normal ventilation in equilibrium and washout images.

The most likely diagnosis is?

   (a) Pulmonary embolism
   (b) Emphysema
   (c) Chest infection
   (d) Congestive heart failure
   (e) Pulmonary artery stenosis

6. A 40-year-old female non-smoker presents with shortness of breath and reduced exercise tolerance. The chest radiograph shows marked lucency in both lower zones with superiorly displaced right horizontal fissure and flattened hemidiaphragm. The upper zones show normal vascularity and lung shadows.

The most likely diagnosis is?

   (a) Centrilobular emphysema
   (b) Alpha-1-antitrypsin deficiency
   (c) Lymphoma
   (d) Hypersensitivity pneumonitis
   (e) Sarcoidosis

7. A 38-year-old man presents with gradually progressive dyspnoea over 2 years. The chest radiograph shows reduced lung volumes with reticular interstitial changes in both lower zones. HRCT show peripheral and basilar reticular opacities with honeycombing and traction bronchiectasis.

The most likely diagnosis is?

(a) Sarcoidosis
(b) Systemic lupus erythematosus
(c) Chronic hypersensitivity pneumonitis
(d) Idiopathic pulmonary fibrosis
(e) Rheumatoid arthritis

8. A 40-year-old man presents shortness of breath after mild smoke inhalation. The chest radiograph shows a right paratracheal soft tissue shadow. The lungs and hila are clear. CT shows a right paratracheal mass in the mediastinum which contains fluid of 10 Hounsfield units. This has well-defined margins and conforms to the shape of surrounding structures without compressing them. No contrast enhancement is seen.

The most likely diagnosis is?

(a) Sarcoidosis
(b) Lymphoma
(c) Metastases from unknown primary
(d) Bronchogenic cyst
(e) Pericardial cyst

9. A 48-year-old female non-smoker presents to the Accident & Emergency Department with acute dyspnoea and chest pain. The chest radiograph shows bilateral basal airspace shadowing. Chest CT shows disuse basal consolidation and air-bronchograms within a background of ground-glass opacity. There is septal thickening and bilateral pleural effusions.

The most likely diagnosis is?

(a) Desquamative interstitial pneumonitis
(b) Lymphocytic interstitial pneumonitis
(c) Acute interstitial pneumonia
(d) Usual interstitial pneumonitis
(e) Cryptogenic organising pneumonia

10. A 70-year-old retired miner presents with shortness of breath for several months. There is no other significant medical history. The chest radiograph shows calcified pleural plaques at both lung bases and bi-basilar interstitial shadowing. CT shows extensive pleural thickening and calcified pleural plaques with bi-basal, peripheral, interstitial shadows and honeycombing. No lymphadenopathy seen.

The most likely diagnosis is?

(a) Tuberculosis
(b) Asbestosis
(c) Silicosis
(d) Empyema
(e) Sarcoidosis

11. A 60-year-old man presents with history of chronic cough. The chest radiograph shows a 5 cm subpleural mass in the right lower lobe. There is a curvilinear opacity from the lower pole of the mass and the mass courses towards the hilum. CT confirms the mass lesion and demonstrates the bronchovascular bundles converging into the mass in a curvilinear fashion. In addition, there are multiple pleural plaques but no lymphadenopathy.

The most likely diagnosis is?

(a) Bronchogenic carcinoma
(b) Rounded atelectasis
(c) Large parenchymal metastasis
(d) Lymphoma
(e) Arteriovenous malformation

12. A 45-year-old woman presents with recurrent episodes of acute exacerbations of dyspnoea. The chest radiograph shows a left hydropneumothorax with large volume lungs and reticular pattern of interstitial opacities. HRCT shows extensive thin-walled cysts throughout the lung parenchyma.

The most likely diagnosis is?

(a) Emphysema
(b) Langerhans cell histiocytosis
(c) Lymphangioleiomyomatosis
(d) Idiopathic pulmonary fibrosis
(e) Neurofibromatosis

13. A 42-year-old female non-smoker presents with recurrent episodes of epistaxis, dyspnoea and occasional haemoptysis. The chest radiograph shows a 3 cm serpiginous nodule in the right mid zone with an apparent draining vessel from the hilum.

The most likely diagnosis is?

(a) Neurilemmoma

(b) Hamartoma

(c) Pulmonary arteriovenous malformation

(d) Adenocarcinoma

(e) Post-primary tuberculosis

14. A 35-year-old pet shop owner presents with shortness of breath. The chest radiograph is normal. HRCT shows diffuse ground-glass centrilobular opacities involving both lungs. No lymphadenopathy is seen.

The most likely diagnosis is:

(a) Sarcoidosis

(b) Pneumoconiosis

(c) Hypersensitivity pneumonitis

(d) Cystic fibrosis

(e) Lymphangioleiomyomatosis

15. A 20-year-old woman is brought to the Accident & Emergency Department by ambulance after being found unresponsive on the street. Examination shows pinpoint pupils and induration in the right groin. The chest radiograph shows bilateral patchy diffuse air space shadowing predominantly in the middle and upper zones with central peribronchial cuffing. No pleural effusion or pneumothorax seen.

The most likely diagnosis is?

(a) Pulmonary oedema secondary to opiate overdose

(b) Acute respiratory distress syndrome

(c) Lung contusion

(d) Renal failure

(e) Fat embolism

16. A 20-year-old woman was admitted with pleuritic chest pain, cough and high fever with a history of intravenous drug abuse. The chest radiograph shows bilateral, multiple lung cavities with both thin and thick walls. Moderate left pleural effusion seen.

    What is the most likely diagnosis?

    (a) Metastatic disease
    (b) Septic pulmonary emboli
    (c) Eosinophilic pneumonia
    (d) Rheumatoid lung
    (e) Bronchitis obliterans organising pneumonia

17. A 37-year-old homosexual man who recently tested positive for HIV presents with cough and shortness of breath. The chest radiograph shows bilateral, thin walled upper lobe cavities and perihilar parenchymal opacities. There is a small right pneumothorax.

    What is the most likely diagnosis?

    (a) Wegener's granulomatosis
    (b) *Pneumocystis jirovecii* infection
    (c) Metastases
    (d) Bronchiectasis
    (e) Bacterial pneumonia

18. A 65-year-old foundry worker presents with cough and progressive shortness of breath. The chest radiograph shows bilateral upper lobe opacities with multiple hilar lymph nodes showing 'egg shell' calcification.

    What is the most likely diagnosis?

    (a) Silicosis
    (b) Sarcoidosis
    (c) Tuberculosis
    (d) Lymphoma
    (e) Metastases

19. A 45-year-old woman with a facial skin discoloration presents with a left-sided hemiparesis. The chest radiograph shows a 2 cm round mass in the left lower lobe. CT confirms the lung mass and shows an enlarged feeding artery and draining vein. No other chest abnormality is seen.

What is the most likely diagnosis?

(a) Small cell lung cancer
(b) Metastasis
(c) Arteriovenous malformation
(d) Tuberculoma
(e) Rheumatoid nodule

20. A 60-year-old patient under treatment for lymphoma presents with chest pain. The chest radiograph and blood results are normal. A V/Q scan shows normal perfusion and patchy areas of ventilation defects in the lungs.

Which of the following is the unlikely diagnosis?

(a) Asthma
(b) Chronic obstructive pulmonary disease
(c) Acute bronchitis
(d) Sarcoidosis
(e) Pulmonary embolism

21. A recently diagnosed HIV-positive man presents with fever and cough. The chest radiograph shows bilateral perihilar interstitial infiltrates and apical ground-glass shadowing. The most likely causative microorganism is?

What is the most likely diagnosis?

(a) *Cryptococcus neoformans*
(b) *Mycobacterium tuberculosis*
(c) *Pneumocystis jirovecii*
(d) *Candida albicans*
(e) *Toxoplasmosis*

22. A 55-year-old woman presents with left-sided ptosis and shoulder pain. The chest radiograph shows a mass in the left lung apex. CT confirms a large superior sulcus tumour eroding through the posterior chest wall and rib.

What is the most likely diagnosis?

(a) Adenocarcinoma

(b) Squamous cell carcinoma

(c) Small cell undifferentiated carcinoma

(d) Undifferentiated large cell carcinoma

(e) Scar carcinoma

23. A 64-year-old non-smoker presents with right chest pain and cough. CT shows a 3 cm spiculated mass in the right upper lobe, abutting the lateral chest wall.

The likely histology is expected to be?

(a) Adenocarcinoma

(b) Squamous cell carcinoma

(c) Small cell undifferentiated carcinoma

(d) Undifferentiated large cell carcinoma

(e) Oat cell cancer

24. An 18-year-old man presents with a history of recurrent chest infections. The chest radiograph shows a left paraspinal soft tissue density behind the heart. Contrast-enhanced CT shows a 6 cm lobulated, multicystic lesion in the left lower lobe containing solid and cystic components. There is a feeding artery from the thoracic aorta into the lesion.

What is the most likely diagnosis?

(a) Extralobar sequestration

(b) Intralobar sequestration

(c) Congenital cystic adenomatoid malformation

(d) Abscess

(e) Lipoid pneumonia

25. A 60-year-old man presents in the accident and emergency department with acute back pain and chest pain. The chest radiograph shows a widened superior mediastinum. CT shows an intimal flap in the ascending aorta with contrast filling on either side of the flap. The arch and descending aorta appear normal.

What is the most likely diagnosis?

(a) Aortic aneurysm

(b) Stanford type B dissection of aorta

(c) DeBakey type I dissection of aorta

(d) DeBakey type II dissection of aorta

(e) DeBakey type III dissection of aorta

26. A 25-year-old man presents with persistent cough. The chest radiograph shows a smoothly marginated opacity in the right cardiophrenic recess. CT shows a 4 cm lesion abutting the pericardium and a small pericardial effusion. The lesion shows no contrast enhancement and contents have Hounsfield units of < 10. On MRI, the abnormality returns uniform high signal intensity on T2-weighted images.

What is the most likely diagnosis?

(a) Pericardial fat pad

(b) Enlarged pericardial lymph nodes

(c) Pericardial cyst

(d) Haematoma

(e) Thymolipoma

27. A 65-year-old man with history of stroke presents with chest pain. The chest radiograph shows a thin curvilinear area of calcification in the lower part of left heart border.

What is the likely site of calcification?

(a) Left atrium

(b) Left ventricle

(c) Right atrium

(d) Left descending coronary artery

(e) Mitral valve

28. A 56-year-old patient with history of cardiac valve replacement presents with acute-onset chest pain. A frontal chest radiograph shows an enlarged heart with laterally displaced left cardiac apex and a metallic ring shadow is seen to be overlapping the spine and horizontally positioned.

Which cardiac valve is this likely to be?

(a) Aortic
(b) Mitral
(c) Tricuspid
(d) Pulmonary
(e) Mitral or aortic

29. A 58-year-old man recently had a cardiac pacemaker. On frontal chest radiograph, the tip of the electrode lies 3 cm medial to the cardiac apex.

What is the most likely site of the electrode tip?

(a) Left atrial appendage
(b) Right atrial appendage
(c) Left ventricle
(d) Right ventricle
(e) Coronary sinus

30. A 46-year-old man presents with fever and cough. A frontal chest radiograph shows loss of the lower part of the left heart border with hazy shadowing in the region.

The most likely site of infection in the lung is?

(a) Lingula
(b) Apicoposterior segment of left upper lobe
(c) Apical segment of left upper lobe
(d) Medial basal segment of left lower lobe
(e) Lateral basal segment of left lower lobe

31. A right-sided subclavian line was inserted in a patient on chemotherapy.

On a frontal chest radiograph, the acceptable position of the tip of the line would be?

(a) Right distal internal jugular vein
(b) Lower part of right heart border
(c) Just above the level of right anterior first intercostal space
(d) Upper part of right heart border, at the level of right hilum
(e) Distal part of right subclavian vein

32. A 35-year-old male smoker with cough shows a 3 cm mass in the right upper lobe. CT confirms the well-defined lesion with smooth margins and calcification and identifies few non-specific lymph nodes in mediastinum. PET–CT shows minimal uptake with SUV < 1.5.

What is the most likely diagnosis?

(a) Hamartoma
(b) Consolidation
(c) Bronchogenic carcinoma
(d) Metastasis
(e) Scarring

33. A 42-year-old woman with a history of stroke presents with bilateral peripheral oedema. The chest radiograph is normal. Contrast-enhanced CT chest shows an ovoid filling defect in the left atrium and appears to be attached to the atrial septum. On MRI, the lesion appears hypointense on T1 and hyperintense on T2.

What is the most likely diagnosis?

(a) Cardiac metastasis
(b) Cardiac lipoma
(c) Left atrial myxoma
(d) Wegener's granulomatosis
(e) Sarcoidosis

34. A 58-year-old man was found to have an incidental lesion measuring 5 cm in the anterior mediastinum. The lesion shows heterogenous enhancement on CT with punctate calcifications. On MRI, the lesion is isointense to muscle, with cystic components and hyperintense on T2.

What is the most likely diagnosis?

(a) Thymolipoma
(b) Thymoma
(c) Lymphoma
(d) Thymic carcinoma
(e) Metastasis

35. A 55-year-old man had a left pneumonectomy for bronchogenic carcinoma. 10 days later, a chest radiograph shows that approximately 50% of the pneumonectomy space is filled with fluid and there is an air-fluid level.

What is the most likely diagnosis?

(a) Bronchopleural fistula

(b) Empyema

(c) Normal evolution of pneumonectomy space

(d) Chylothorax

(e) Post-pneumonectomy syndrome

36. A 62-year-old smoker presents with haemoptysis. The chest radiograph shows a mass in right paracardiac region with loss of right heart border.

The lesion is most likely to be in?

(a) Right middle lobe

(b) Apical segment of right lower lobe

(c) Posterior segment of right upper lobe

(d) Medial basal segment of right lower lobe

(e) Anterior basal segment of right lower lobe

37. A 46-year-old woman with a history of breast cancer presents with persistent cough. The chest radiograph shows reticular shadowing in the left lower zone. HRCT shows diffuse septal thickening and nodularity in the left lower lobe.

What is the most likely diagnosis?

(a) Heart failure

(b) Lymphangitic carcinomatosis

(c) Sarcoidosis

(d) Amyloidosis

(e) Respiratory bronchiolitis

38. A 62-year-old man with history of stroke and swallowing difficulties presents with persistent cough. HRCT shows patchy areas of bilateral 'tree-in-bud' pattern in the lower lobes.

What is the most likely diagnosis?

(a) Sarcoidosis

(b) Miliary tuberculosis

(c) Chronic aspiration

(d) Hypersensitivity pneumonitis

(e) Langerhans cell granulomatosis

39. A 32-year-old man presents with cough. The chest radiographs shows a 4 cm paraspinal mass lesion. CT chest demonstrates a smooth, well-defined dumbbell shaped mass in the left paravertebral region. The lesion expands the neural foramen and extends into the spinal canal.

What is the most likely diagnosis?

(a) Neuroblastoma
(b) Neurofibroma
(c) Bronchogenic carcinoma
(d) Lymphoma
(e) Extramedullary haematopoiesis

40. A 60-year-old recently retired postman presents with chronic cough. The chest radiograph shows soft tissue opacity extending from the right hilum to the lateral chest wall, with loss of the right heart border. There is loss of right lung volume and the right costophrenic angle is seen. Bronchoscopy demonstrates a large endobronchial mass.

What is the most likely bronchus involved?

(a) Right upper lobe bronchus
(b) Right middle lobe bronchus
(c) Right lower lobe bronchus
(d) Bronchus intermedius
(e) Right lower lobe apical segment bronchus

41. A 40-year-old man with a history of intravenous drug abuse presents with back pain. CT shows an infrarenal aortic aneurysm and left psoas abscess.

What is the most likely finding on CT?

(a) Lobulated, saccular aneurysm
(b) Fusiform aneurysm
(c) Pseudoaneurysm
(d) Periaortic gas
(e) Extensive mural thrombus

42. A 64-year-old man presents with a history of chronic cough and chest pain. The chest radiograph shows a 2 cm soft tissue lesion in the left upper zone with a crescent shaped gas collection around. CT shows a dependent 2 cm round mass in a cavity.

What is the most likely diagnosis?

(a) Wegener's granulomatosis

(b) Aspergilloma

(c) Lung abscess

(d) Rheumatoid nodule

(e) Metastasis

43. A 62-year-old man with known primary malignancy presents with haemoptysis. Chest radiograph shows a cavitating lesion in the left mid zone.

Which is the least likely diagnosis?

(a) Carcinoma of the colon

(b) Melanoma

(c) Transitional cell carcinoma of the bladder

(d) Carcinoma of the prostate

(e) Squamous cell carcinoma of the lung

44. A 36-year-old man presents with cough and haemoptysis. The chest radiograph demonstrates a 4 cm mass lesion in right upper lobe with calcifications. CT-guided biopsy shows that the lesion is malignant.

What is the most unlikely primary?

(a) Osteosarcoma femur

(b) Thyroid carcinoma

(c) Testicular primary

(d) Carcinoma colon

(e) Lymphoma

45. A 64-year-old woman known to have chronic rheumatoid arthritis presents with shortness of breath.

The most common feature seen on the chest radiograph is?

(a) Pleural effusion

(b) Rheumatoid nodule

(c) Diffuse interstitial fibrosis

(d) Bronchiectasis

(e) Pericardial effusion

46. An 18-year-old man was brought to the Accident & Emergency Department. The patient was the driver of a car involved in a road traffic accident.

What is the most common/expected abnormality on chest CT?

(a) Pneumothorax

(b) Flail chest

(c) Clavicle fracture

(d) Diaphragmatic injury

(e) Oesophageal rupture

47. A 45-year-old woman had allogenic bone marrow transplant for treatment of leukaemia. Two weeks later she developed cough and shortness of breath. CT demonstrates bilateral ground-glass shadowing, thickened interstitial lines and bilateral pleural effusion.

What is the most likely diagnosis?

(a) Bronchiolitis obliterans

(b) Drug toxicity

(c) Pulmonary oedema

(d) Diffuse alveolar haemorrhage

(e) Bronchiolitis obliterans organising pneumonia

48. A 68-year-old man presents with a history of chronic cough. The chest radiograph shows a diffuse reticular nodular pattern with mid-lower zone predominance. HRCT shows a symmetrical reticular pattern with sub-pleural honeycombing and traction bronchiectasis.

What is the most likely diagnosis?

(a) Sarcoidosis

(b) Hypersensitivity pneumonitis

(c) Idiopathic pulmonary fibrosis

(d) Asbestosis

(e) Silicosis

49. A 35-year-old man presents with cough. Chest radiograph shows a low volume right lung and a gently curving tubular shadow coursing from the lower part of right inferior pulmonary artery towards the right costovertebral angle. The shadow widens as it descends towards the diaphragm.

What is the most likely diagnosis?

(a) Pulmonary sequestration
(b) Scimitar syndrome
(c) Wandering vein
(d) Swyer–James syndrome
(e) Chronic pulmonary thromboembolism

50. A 38-year-old bird keeper presents with recurrent episodes of flu-like symptoms. The chest radiograph is normal. HRCT shows extensive bilateral symmetrical, small ill-defined centrilobular nodules.

What is the most likely diagnosis?

(a) Sarcoidosis
(b) Idiopathic pulmonary fibrosis
(c) Scleroderma
(d) Hypersensitivity pneumonitis
(e) Respiratory bronchiolitis–interstitial lung disease

ANSWERS

1. **(b) Asbestosis**

    All the other given options are known to cause egg shell calcification of the hilar lymph nodes.

2. **(b) 0.5 mL of 1:1000 of adrenaline intramuscular injection**

    This is the recommended dose in cases of anaphylactic contrast reaction as recommended by the Royal College of Radiologists.

3. **(e) Scleroderma**

    Other conditions cause predominantly upper zone disease.

4. **(b) Sarcoidosis**

    Garland's triad, seen in sarcoidosis, involves bilateral hilar nodes and paratracheal lymph nodes. Seventy per cent of cases of sarcoidosis have elevated serum levels of angiotensin-converting enzyme.

5. **(a) Pulmonary embolism**

    This is the most likely diagnosis. If multiple ventilation-perfusion defects are seen in areas where there are no corresponding chest radiographic abnormalities, pulmonary embolism is highly probable. Rarely, vasculitis can produce such appearance, but the patient's clinical history and presentation should allow accurate diagnosis.

6. **(b) Alpha-1-antitrypsin deficiency**

    Patients with this condition develop severe panacinar emphysema with basilar predominance due to gravitational distribution of pulmonary blood flow. On CT, the margins of cysts are poorly visualised due to involvement of the entire secondary lobule. This pattern is significantly different from chronic smoker's emphysema, which tends to develop centrilobular emphysema with upper zone predominance and cysts with well-defined margins.

7. **(d) Idiopathic pulmonary fibrosis**

    These are typical radiographic and HRCT features of idiopathic pulmonary fibrosis.

8. **(d) Bronchogenic cyst**

    These are developmental cysts that are a part of bronchopulmonary foregut malformations. These often have a fibrous capsule and filled with fluid attenuation mucoid material. They do not cause any mass effect and conforms to the shape of surrounding mediastinal structures. On MRI, they are bright on T2 but due to protein content, the signal on T1 is variable. No contrast enhancement is seen.

9. **(c) Acute interstitial pneumonia**

    This clinically presents as adult respiratory distress syndrome and has high mortality. It has a fulminant course leading to respiratory failure and requiring mechanical ventilation with a mortality of > 50%. CT findings are non-specific but include bilateral, diffuse ground-glass opacity with consolidation and air bronchograms. Honeycombing and traction bronchiectasis may be seen in advanced cases after recovery.

10. **(b) Asbestosis**

    This is defined as interstitial pulmonary fibrosis in association with asbestos exposure (pleural plaques and calcification). Disease progression is from bases to apices and honeycombing is seen later in the disease. Lymphadenopathy is usually absent, and its presence should suggest alternate diagnosis

11. **(b) Round atelectasis**

    Also called 'folded lung' or 'asbestos pseudotumour'. The lesion forms acute angles with the pleura indicating its parenchymal location. Pleural thickening is usually an associated finding. It usually affects the lower lobes and there is volume loss. The characteristic sign of round atelectasis is the 'comet tail' sign. As the lung collapses, the bronchovascular bundle is pulled into the region. As they reach the mass they diverge and arch around the surface to merge with the inferior pole of the mass. This is typically well demonstrated on CT.

12. **(c) Lymphangioleiomyomatosis**

    Exclusively seen in women of childbearing age, characterised by large lungs, coarse interstitial pattern, extensive lung cysts and recurrent pneumo- or chylopneumothorax.

    In histiocytosis, cysts are seen in the upper two-thirds of the lung with sparing of the costophrenic angle, cysts are variable in thickness, and there is septal thickening. Idiopathic pulmonary fibrosis show irregular thick-walled peripheral cysts and honeycombing. Neurofibromatosis has cysts in apical location. Emphysema shows imperceptible cyst walls; cysts show segmental distribution, lobular architecture preserved with the bronchovascular bundle in a central position.

13. (c) Pulmonary arteriovenous malformation

70% of pulmonary arteriovenous malformations are associated with Osler–Weber–Rendu syndrome also called hereditary hemorrhagic telangiectasia (HHT) which is associated with multiorgan arteriovenous malformations. A patient with HHT may present with epistaxis, GI bleeding, skin telangiectasia etc. Chest radiography shows a sharply demarcated mass, typically round or oval, and feeding vessels can be seen from the hilum. Contrast-enhanced CT chest confirms abnormal communication between pulmonary arteries and pulmonary veins.

14. (c) Hypersensitivity pneumonitis

HRCT appearances are typical of subacute hypersensitivity pneumonitis. This is caused by inhalation of antigenic organic particles. The subacute phase is characterised by intermittent exposure to antigens with symptoms arising over weeks to months. The chronic phase is characterised by the presence of fibrosis.

15. (a) Pulmonary oedema secondary to opiate overdose

Pin point pupils and right groin infection suggests intravenous drug abuser. Radiographic findings of non-cardiogenic pulmonary oedema are non-central, extensive, patchy, bilateral airspace shadowing with indistinct vessels and peribronchial cuffing.

Cardiogenic oedema is characterised by cardiac enlargement, pleural effusions, upper lobe venous diversion, Kerley-B lines and peribronchial cuffing.

16. (b) Septic pulmonary emboli

Given the history of intravenous drug abuse, multiple lung cavities are likely to be secondary to septic pulmonary emboli.

Eosinophilic pneumonia and bronchitis obliterans organising pneumonia are unlikely to cause cavitation.

17. (b) *Pneumocystis jirovecii* pneumonia

Pneumocystis jirovecii pneumonia (previously called *Pneumocystis carinii* pneumonia) is seen in HIV positive individuals. Pneumatocoeles are seen in 10% of cases and some may progress to develop a pneumothorax.

18. (a) Silicosis

This appearance can be seen in both silicosis and sarcoidosis; however, given the occupational history, silicosis is the favoured diagnosis.

Treated lymphoma can also give egg shell calcification.

19. (c) Arteriovenous malformation (AVM)

Patients with AVM present with cough, haemoptysis or occasionally with cerebral embolism. Fifty per cent of pulmonary AVMs are associated with Osler–Weber–Rendu disease (many have AVMs elsewhere, including the skin, mucous membranes and other organs).

20. (e) Pulmonary embolism is the unlikely diagnosis

Pulmonary embolism will demonstrate abnormal perfusion defects with or without ventilation defects

21. (c) *Pneumocystis jirovecii*

This organism is the commonest cause of chest infection in patients with AIDS. It usually has an insidious onset with bilateral perihilar infiltrates. There may also be diffuse bilateral alveolar infiltrates and ground-glass shadowing. Patients on prophylactic aerosolized pentamidine may show an apical predominance.

22. (b) Squamous cell carcinoma

Superior sulcal tumours are frequently squamous cell carcinomas. They may lead to atrophy of muscles secondary to brachial plexus involvement or/and Horner's syndrome secondary to involvement of sympathetic chain and stellate ganglion.

23. (a) Adenocarcinoma

Adenocarcinoma is the most common type associated with non-smokers and is usually seen in the periphery.

Squamous cell carcinoma, small cell undifferentiated type and undifferentiated large cell cancers are strongly associated with smoking.

24. (b) Intralobar sequestration

These are the typical features of an intralobar sequestration.

Extralobar sequestration often is seen usually before 6 months age and associated with other congenital anomalies. The other causes listed do not have any feeding vessels.

25. (d) DeBakey type II dissection of aorta

This type involves only the ascending thoracic aorta and is surgically repaired.

26. (c) Pericardial cyst

These are usually incidental finding and contain fluid. A level of < 10 Hounsfield units is typical.

Pericardial fat pad and thymolipoma would show fat on CT with lower Hounsfield units.

27. (b) Left ventricle

This is the typical site for left ventricular calcifications.

Valvular calcifications are located within the heart. Coronary artery calcifications are seen along the upper part of left heart border and have a 'tram-track' appearance.

28. (a) Aortic valve

The aortic and mitral valves are seen adjacent to the spine and can be difficult to separate. However, the aortic valve is usually seen horizontally situated while the mitral valve is generally situated vertically. On a lateral projection, if a line is drawn from the carina to the anterior costophrenic angle, the aortic valve lies above this line and the mitral valve below it.

29. (d) Right ventricle

The tip of the ventricular lead is seen at the apex of right ventricle.

30. (a) Lingula

The lingular segment in the left lung lies adjacent to the heart and collapse/ consolidation in this segment leads to loss of the lower part of left heart border.

31. (d) Upper part of right heart border, at the level of right hilum

The tip of the subclavian line must be distal to the valves and in the superior vena cava. The last valves in the subclavian and internal jugular veins are 2.0–2.5 cm proximal to their union. The brachiocephalic vein and superior vena cava do not contain valves.

The superior vena cava commences at the level of right first intercostal space and tip of lines above this lie in the distal internal jugular vein. A catheter tip in right atrium or right ventricle may cause arrhythmias.

32. (a) Hamartoma

This is the most common benign tumour of the lung. It commonly contains calcification and fat (diagnostic). On a PET scan, hamartomas usually show poor uptake while the other listed conditions may show high uptake on PET.

33. (c) Left atrial myxoma

Embolisation may lead to strokes in patients with left atrial myxoma.

Wegener's and sarcoidosis in the heart are very rare. Lipoma shows fat density and signal on imaging.

34. (b) Thymoma

Thymolipoma are rare, predominantly fat-containing neoplasms.

Lymphoma presents with extensive lymph node masses in the mediastinum.

35. (c) Normal evolution of pneumonectomy space

After 7–10 days, approximately half to two-thirds of the pneumonectomy space fills up with fluid. Complete filling with fluid is seen in 2–4 months. A small amount of air may be seen indefinitely. Post-pneumonectomy syndrome is seen after 1 year.

Bronchopleural fistula should be considered if there is persistent pneumothorax or if the air–fluid level drops by > 2 cm or there is reappearance of air in a previously opacified pneumonectomy space.

36. (a) Right middle lobe

The right middle lobe lies adjacent to the right heart border and disease of the right middle lobe (e.g. collapse/consolidation) results in loss of normal sharp outline of the right heart order.

37. (b) Lymphangitic carcinomatosis

Given the history of malignancy, septal thickening with septal nodularity is suggestive/suspicious of lymphangitic carcinomatosis.

38. (c) Chronic aspiration

Given the history of swallowing difficulties and stroke, the patient is likely to have aspiration pneumonitis presenting as a result of severe bronchiolar impaction with clubbing of the distal bronchioles.

39. (b) Neurofibroma

Neurofibromas are typically dumbbell shaped and extend into the spinal canal with expansion of the neural foramen.

Neuroblastoma is seen usually in children, are heterogenous tumours and show calcification. Bronchogenic carcinoma causes bony destruction and lymphoma rarely has isolated posterior mediastinal mass.

40. **(d) Bronchus intermedius**

    The chest radiograph findings are suggestive of combined right middle lobe and right lower lobe collapse secondary to tumour obstructing the bronchus intermedius.

41. **(a) Lobulated, saccular aneurysm**

    The patient is likely to have a mycotic aortic aneurysm. Mycotic aneurysms are commonly saccular and lobulated and less commonly fusiform. They may be associated with psoas abscess, discitis or osteomyelitis.

42. **(b) Aspergilloma**

    CT halo sign is characteristic for aspergilloma where a dependent, rounded nodule is seen in a cavity or a cyst. Prone and supine CT demonstrates mobility of mycetoma in the cavity.

43. **(d) Carcinoma of the prostate**

    The rest of the tumours are all common causes of cavitating metastatic lesions.

44. **(e) Lymphoma**

    Lymphoma lesions do not usually show calcifications unless there is a history of treatment with radiation.

    The rest of the tumours listed can present with calcifying lung metastatic deposits.

45. **(a) Pleural effusion**

    This is the most common finding on a chest radiograph in patients with chronic rheumatoid arthritis, seen in more than 90% cases.

46. **(a) Pneumothorax**

    Pneumothorax, lung contusions and rib fractures are the most common expected abnormalities in blunt trauma to chest, seen in more than two-thirds of cases.

    Other abnormalities are far less common.

47. **(c) Pulmonary oedema**

    This is usually secondary to fluid overload and associated renal dysfunction.

    Bronchiolitis obliterans and bronchiolitis obliterans organising pneumonia are late complications seen after 3 months. Drug toxicity and alveolar haemorrhages may present with ground-glass shadowing but do not show pleural effusions or interstitial involvement.

48. (c) Idiopathic pulmonary fibrosis

These radiographic and HRCT appearances are typically a feature of idiopathic pulmonary fibrosis.

Sarcoidosis affects upper zones predominantly. Hypersensitivity pneumonitis usually spares extreme bases but sometimes may be difficult to separate from idiopathic pulmonary fibrosis. Asbestosis also may show peripheral honeycombing but is associated with pleural plaques.

49. (b) Scimitar syndrome

Also called congenital pulmonary venolobar syndrome. There is congenital hypoplasia of the right lung with anomalous pulmonary venous drainage into the inferior vena cava. The anomalous vein seen best on radiographs and CT reconstructions, is shaped like a Turkish sword (scimitar sign). The right lung is almost exclusively involved.

50. (d) Hypersensitivity pneumonitis

Given the history of bird keeping, and diffuse centrilobular shadowing in the lungs, the diagnosis is likely to be hypersensitivity pneumonitis.

Chapter 2

Musculoskeletal system and trauma

QUESTIONS

1. A 45-year-old man attends the Accident & Emergency Department with a 1-week history of foot pain. He is a regular runner and recently completed the London marathon. There is a history of lymphoma 15 years ago treated with chemotherapy. He is also diabetic and has chronic renal failure. Radiographs demonstrated a subtle periosteal reaction at the second metatarsal shaft. Bone scan shows focal tracer uptake in the second metatarsal region.

    What is the most likely diagnosis?

    (a) Lymphoma deposit in second metatarsal
    (b) Stress fracture
    (c) Osteomyelitis
    (d) Neuropathic foot
    (e) Osteomalacia

2. A 55-year-old housewife attended her GP with a gradually growing soft tissue swelling on the dorsum of her foot for 1 year. The swelling is tender and mobile in a side-to-side direction. Ultrasound shows a 4 cm hypervascular lesion on the dorsum of the foot between the tendons of extensor hallucis and extensor digitorum. MRI shows that the lesion is bright on STIR and intermediate signal on T1. It shows homogenous enhancement with gadolinium.

    What is the most likely diagnosis?

    (a) Soft tissue ganglion
    (b) Peripheral nerve sheath tumour
    (c) Lipoma
    (d) Liposarcoma
    (e) Callus from a previous fracture.

3. A 34-year-old sedentary male office worker presents with a 2-month history of heel pain. A radiograph demonstrates a well-defined lytic lesion in the calcaneum. This produces mild expansion with endosteal scalloping and has a central ossified nodule. On MRI, the lesion is high signal on T1 and T2.

    What is the most likely diagnosis?

    (a) Giant cell tumour
    (b) Fibrous cortical defect
    (c) Intraosseous lipoma
    (d) Osteoid osteoma
    (e) Solitary bone cyst

4. A 10-year-old boy presented with fracture of the left proximal humerus sustained during a tackle in a football match. Plain radiographs show a pathological fracture and underlying lytic lesion in the metaphysis of the proximal humerus. The lesion shows endosteal scalloping and a small bone fragment in the floor of the cyst. MRI features include intermediate signal on T1 and high signal on T2 with a fluid–fluid level.

    What is the most likely diagnosis of the underlying bony lesion?

    (a) Unicameral bone cyst
    (b) Lymphoma
    (c) Aneurysmal bone cyst
    (d) Telangiectatic osteosarcoma
    (e) Giant cell tumour

5. A 15-year-old boy attended the Accident & Emergency Department with ankle pain after a twisting injury 7 days previously. The history suggests there has been ill-defined swelling and ache for a few weeks. The plain radiograph shows a fracture in the distal fibula, with lamellar periosteal reaction. There appears to be an associated soft tissue bulge.

    What is the most likely diagnosis?

    (a) Fracture with large haematoma
    (b) Neuroblastoma metastasis
    (c) Lymphoma
    (d) Ewing's sarcoma with fracture
    (e) Osteomyelitis

6. An 80-year-old diabetic complains of left groin pain. He undergoes twice a week haemodialysis. The plain radiograph shows large globular periarticular calcifications around both hip joints. A bone scan shows absence of renal activity and 'superscan' appearance. The calcifications also show increased tracer uptake.

The most likely cause of the calcifications is?

(a) Dermatomyositis
(b) Renal osteodystrophy
(c) Scleroderma
(d) Calcium pyrophosphate deposition disease.
(e) Renal osteodystrophy

7. A 65-year-old woman with chronic rheumatoid arthritis, had fracture of the lateral malleolus which was treated by a cast immobilisation. Since removal of the plaster, the foot has been swollen and painful on movements. Plain radiographs show that the fracture is united but the bones show diffuse osteopenia with endosteal scalloping and severe periarticular demineralisation. Bone scan shows increased uptake on three phase scintigram.

The most likely cause of the patient's symptoms is?

(a) Reflex sympathetic dystrophy
(b) Transient regional osteoporosis
(c) Myelomatosis
(d) Infection
(e) Disuse osteoporosis

8. A 40-year-old woman with lung cancer and multiple liver metastases presents with back pain and left L5 radiculopathy. Plain radiography demonstrates prominent vertical striations in L4 vertebral body. MRI scans demonstrated a sequestrated disc pressing the left L5 nerve root in the lateral recess. The L4 vertebral body shows a well-defined lesion, returning high signal on T1 and T2.

The lesion in the L4 vertebral body is?

(a) Intraosseous ganglion
(b) Metastatic deposit from lung cancer
(c) Haemangioma
(d) Osteoid osteoma
(e) Schmorl's node

9. A 20-year-old athlete presented with chronic leg pain relieved with aspirin. The plain radiograph shows 2–3 cm area of sclerosis and cortical thickening in the midshaft tibia. CT shows a 1 cm lytic lesion with central mineralisation. MRI demonstrates a bone oedema pattern but normal surrounding soft tissues.

    The most likely cause of underlying pathology is?

    (a) Stress fracture
    (b) Ewing's sarcoma
    (c) Osteomyelitis
    (d) Enchondroma
    (e) Osteoid osteoma

10. A 40-year-old mother presents with knee pain. Plain radiographs show an eccentric, expansile, lytic lesion with a narrow zone of transition in the lateral femoral condyle extending to subarticular bone. The lateral cortex is thinned but no periosteal reaction or sclerosis is seen. MRI shows a well-defined bony lesion with intermediate signal on T1 and mixed signal on T2 and multiple fluid–fluid levels.

    The most likely diagnosis is?

    (a) Benign fibrous histiocytoma
    (b) Giant cell tumour
    (c) Telangiectatic osteosarcoma
    (d) Brodie's abscess
    (e) Simple bone cyst

11. A 10-year-old white boy presented with mass in abdomen and bilateral hip pain. He was found to have splenomegaly and pancytopaenia. Pelvic radiograph suggests bilateral avascular necrosis of femoral heads. MRI shows diffuse low signal bone marrow on T1 and T2.

    What is the most likely diagnosis?

    (a) Gaucher's disease
    (b) Sickle cell disease
    (c) Perthes' disease
    (d) Leukaemia
    (e) Multifocal histiocytosis

12. A 40-year-old man presents with right knee pain. Plain radiography shows a large joint effusion. MRI of the knee shows multiple foci of low signal intensity seen in the synovium on T1, T2 and gradient-echo sequences. There is a moderate joint effusion.

The most likely diagnosis is?

(a) Haemangioma
(b) Pigmented villonodular synovitis
(c) Rheumatoid arthritis
(d) Synovial sarcoma
(e) Synovial chondromatosis

13. A 55-year-old man presents with pain and swelling in the left big toe. The plain radiograph shows periarticular erosions with sclerotic margins and overhanging edges in the first metatarsophalangeal joint. The joint space is preserved and there is moderate surrounding soft tissue swelling.

The most likely diagnosis is?

(a) Rheumatoid arthritis
(b) Erosive osteoarthritis
(c) Gouty arthritis
(d) Psoriatic arthropathy
(e) Calcium pyrophosphate deposition disease.

14. A 40-year-old chronic smoker with recently diagnosed bronchogenic carcinoma presents with bilateral leg pains. A plain radiograph shows lamellar periosteal reaction in bilateral tibia. A bone scan demonstrates diffusely increased uptake along the cortical margins of the tibial diaphysis.

The most likely diagnosis is?

(a) Bilateral tibial metastases
(b) Osteomyelitis
(c) Chronic venous stasis
(d) Hypertrophic osteoarthropathy
(e) Acromegaly

15. An elderly patient with history of urinary frequency and dribbling presents with right hip pain. A radiograph of pelvis shows there is marked thickening of the iliopectineal line with acetabular protrusion, coarsening of the trabecular pattern and increased sclerosis in the entire right hemipelvis. The left hemipelvis appears normal.

The most likely diagnosis is?

(a) Sclerotic metastases from prostate carcinoma
(b) Paget's disease
(c) Lymphoma
(d) Normal variant
(e) Fluorosis

16. A 35-year-old man presents with knee pain. MRI shows a 1.5 cm homogenous ovoid lesion which pushes the medial collateral ligament. It returns high signal on STIR and T2 images. There is also a horizontal cleavage tear of the posterior horn of the medial meniscus and a radial tear of the lateral meniscus.

The most likely cause of the lesion is?

(a) Dissecting bakers cyst
(b) Ganglion
(c) Pes anserinus bursa
(d) Haemangioma
(e) Meniscal cyst

17. A 21-year-old man presents with multiple swellings and focal areas of bluish discoloration in both hands. Plain radiograph of the hands show multiple, well-defined, expanded lytic lesions in the metacarpals. These lesions show stippled calcifications in the matrix and cause cortical thinning. Multiple small round calcifications are seen in the surrounding soft tissues.

The most likely diagnosis is?

(a) Ollier's disease
(b) Maffucci's syndrome
(c) Metastases
(d) Diaphyseal aclasis
(e) Kaposi's sarcoma

18. An 80-year-old woman complains of pain in both hands. Radiography of the hands shows bilateral central articular 'seagull' erosions affecting the interphalangeal joints of fingers in both hands. Mild periarticular osteoporosis is seen.

The most likely diagnosis is?

(a) Osteoarthritis
(b) Erosive osteoarthritis
(c) Calcium pyrophosphate deposition disease
(d) Gouty arthropathy
(e) Rheumatoid arthritis

19. A 35-year-old woman with moderate hallux valgus deformity, complains of pain between the second and third toes of left foot. Ultrasound shows a 1 cm hypoechoic lesion in the region of the distal intermetatarsal heads of the second and third toes. This is non-compressible and shows no significant vascularity.

The most likely diagnosis is?

(a) Bursitis
(b) Morton's neuroma
(c) Ganglion from metatarsophalangeal joint
(d) Tenosynovitis from the flexor tendons
(e) Synovial sarcoma

20. A 67-year-old man with history of lung cancer and renal transplant had a bone scan. There are multiple focal areas of increased tracer uptake in the left ribs, arranged in a linear pattern. Increased tracer uptake is also identified along the cortices of both humerus and radius bones bilaterally. No renal uptake is seen.

The most likely diagnosis for this appearance is?

(a) Hypertrophic osteoarthropathy with rib metastases
(b) Hypertrophic osteoarthropathy with rib fractures
(c) Normal uptake in lower limbs with rib fractures
(d) Normal uptake in lower limbs with rib metastases
(e) Diffuse skeletal metastases

21. A 60-year-old man with history of diabetes, chronic renal failure and bilateral intermittent claudication, had a left ankle injury 6 months ago. It was treated by open reduction and internal fixation of the medial and lateral malleoli. He now complains of persistent pain and swelling in the ankle and foot. Plain radiographs show marked osteopenia of the bones in the left ankle and foot. Bone scan shows diffuse increased tracer uptake in the periarticular distribution in left ankle and foot.

The likely cause of the bone scan appearances is?

  (a) Chronic ischemic feet

  (b) Hypertrophic osteoarthropathy

  (c) Secondary hyperparathyroidism

  (d) Reflex sympathetic dystrophy

  (e) Diabetic foot

22. A 75-year-old woman presents with symptoms of headache, right leg pain and raised serum alkaline phosphatase. Plain radiography of the right leg shows cortical thickening of the proximal tibia with coarse trabeculations and bowing. A bone scan demonstrates intense tracer uptake in the calvarium and the right tibia.

The most likely diagnosis is?

  (a) Multiple myeloma

  (b) Paget's disease

  (c) Secondary hyperparathyroidism

  (d) Hypertrophic pulmonary osteoarthropathy

  (e) Myelofibrosis

23. A 60-year-old woman with recent history of falls presents with bilateral hip and low back pain. MRI of the pelvis shows bilateral sacral ala fractures and parasymphysial pubic fractures with marginal sclerosis. There is increased tracer uptake on bone scan of these regions.

The most likely diagnosis is?

  (a) Multiple myeloma with pathological fractures

  (b) Insufficiency fractures

  (c) Traumatic fractures

  (d) Metastatic disease with unknown primary

  (e) Lymphoma

24. A 24-year-old man was involved in a road traffic accident. CT of the left knee shows isolated 5 mm depression of the lateral tibial plateau.

    What is the Schatzker classification of this fracture?

    (a) Type 1
    (b) Type 2
    (c) Type 3
    (d) Type 4
    (e) Type 5

25. A 13-year-old footballer complains of pain in the right groin after a tackle. Radiograph of the pelvis shows an avulsion fracture of the lesser tuberosity.

    Which muscle is attached to the lesser tuberosity?

    (a) Iliopsoas
    (b) Rectus femoris
    (c) Sartorius
    (d) Biceps femoris
    (e) Vastus medialis

26. A 10-year-old boy presents after falling down stairs and sustaining injury to his left forearm. Radiographs show a displaced fracture of the proximal shaft ulna and anterior dislocation of the radial head.

    What is the diagnosis?

    (a) Galeazzi fracture dislocation
    (b) Monteggia fracture dislocation
    (c) Essex–Lopresti fracture complex
    (d) Weber fracture
    (e) Maisonneuve fracture

27. A 30-year-old African man presents with knee pain. Radiograph shows a serpiginous area of lucency with sclerotic margins in the proximal metaphysis of tibia. MRI shows a 'double-line' sign on T2-weighted images. There is a linear area of low signal peripheral to a high signal intensity inner border. A bone scan shows no uptake in the area.

    The most likely diagnosis is?

    (a) Bone infarct
    (b) Osteomyelitis
    (c) Enchondroma
    (d) Non-ossifying fibroma
    (e) Osteonecrosis

28. A 62-year-old man presents with sudden-onset pain after minor injury. Plain radiograph shows subchondral sclerosis in the medial femoral condyle and joint effusion. MRI shows a diffuse oedema in the subchondral bone of medial femoral condyle with a crescentic linear fracture in a subchondral location.

The most likely diagnosis is?

(a) Spontaneous osteonecrosis of knee
(b) Osteoarthritis
(c) Osteochondritis desiccans
(d) Calcium pyrophosphate deposition disease
(e) Gout

29. An 18-year-old man presents with progressive swelling of right knee. Radiographs show large joint effusion in the suprapatellar pouch. MRI shows marked synovial thickening and large synovial fronds which return high signal on T1, T2 and proton density images. The lesions are low signal on STIR images.

The most likely diagnosis is?

(a) Synovial lipoma
(b) Synovial osteochondromatosis
(c) Hypertrophic synovitis
(d) Pigmented villonodular synovitis
(e) Lipoma arborescens

30. A 51-year-old man with a palpable nodule on the planter aspect of the foot. Ultrasound shows a 2 cm, vascular and hypoechoic lesion within the mid part of the plantar fascia.

The most likely diagnosis is?

(a) Plantar lipoma
(b) Plantar fibromatosis
(c) Ganglion cyst
(d) Accessory muscle
(e) Haemangioma

31. A 35-year-old woman presents with swelling in the thigh. The radiograph shows a bony excrescence from the femoral cortex without medullary continuity. On MRI there is a soft tissue surrounding the bony excrescence, which returns high signal on T1 and T2 and homogenous low signal on STIR.

    The most likely diagnosis is?

    (a) Osteochondroma
    (b) Osteosarcoma
    (c) Liposarcoma
    (d) Parosteal lipoma
    (e) Intramuscular lipoma

32. A 12-year-old boy presents with a hard lump around his right knee. A radiograph shows a bony projection from the medial part of the tibial metaphysis with continuity of the cortex and medulla of the tibia.

    What is the most likely diagnosis?

    (a) Osteochondroma
    (b) Parosteal osteosarcoma
    (c) Chondrosarcoma
    (d) Periosteal osteosarcoma
    (e) Juxtacortical myositis ossificans

33. A 20-year-old woman presents with pain after injury to the index finger. The radiograph shows a 2 cm lytic lesion with a matrix containing calcifications. There is endosteal scalloping of the cortex with cortical expansion, but no cortical breach.

    The most likely diagnosis is?

    (a) Bone infarct
    (b) Enchondroma
    (c) Chondrosarcoma
    (d) Juxtacortical chondroma
    (e) Epidermoid cyst

34. A 26-year-old man presents with dull pain in the left thigh not relieved with salicylates. Radiograph shows a 3 cm expansile lytic lesion in the mid-shaft of the left femur, which shows reactive sclerosis and periosteal reaction. The bone scan shows intense tracer uptake.

    The most likely diagnosis is?

    (a) Osteoid osteoma
    (b) Osteoblastoma
    (c) Osteosarcoma
    (d) Osteomyelitis
    (e) Aneurysmal bone cyst

35. A 33-year-old man presents with a 2-year history of a hard lump on the left middle finger. A radiograph shows a 2 cm, well-defined, round, densely sclerotic lesion attached to the cortex of the proximal phalanx of the left middle finger. No cortical erosion or periosteal reaction is seen. A bone scan shows no tracer uptake.

    The most likely diagnosis is?

    (a) Enostosis
    (b) Osteoma
    (c) Parosteal osteosarcoma
    (d) Osteochondroma
    (e) Myositis ossificans

36. A 20-year-old football player presents after injuring his right knee in a tackle. Plain radiographs show fracture of the tibial spine with lipohaemarthrosis.

    What structure is attached to the medial part of the anterior tibial spine?

    (a) Anterior cruciate ligament
    (b) Posterior cruciate ligament
    (c) Medial collateral ligament
    (d) Lateral collateral ligament
    (e) Medial meniscus

37. A 40-year-old man with a history of dislocated left hip in a road traffic accident 2 years ago presents with left hip pain. Radiography show flattening and sclerosis in the superolateral part of the femoral head.

The most likely diagnosis is?

(a) Degenerative arthritis
(b) Calcium pyrophosphate deposition disease
(c) Avascular necrosis
(d) Paget's disease
(e) Prostatic metastases

38. A 60-year-old presents with left groin pain. Ultrasound shows a 2 cm hypoechoic lesion bulging medial to the epigastric vessels on Valsalva manoeuvre and absent on rest.

What is the most likely diagnosis?

(a) Direct inguinal hernia
(b) Indirect inguinal hernia
(c) Obturator hernia
(d) Spigelian hernia
(e) Femoral hernia

39. A 40-year-old man presents with right groin pain. Ultrasound shows a 3 cm echogenic soft tissue mass distending the right inguinal canal on straining, and which goes away on relaxation.

What is the most likely diagnosis?

(a) Direct inguinal hernia
(b) Indirect inguinal hernia
(c) Femoral hernia
(d) Obturator hernia
(e) Lymph node

40. A 40-year-old man presents with a lump in the right groin 2 months after a laparoscopic inguinal hernia repair. Ultrasound shows a well-defined homogenous, hyperechoic, avascular soft tissue mass lateral to the inferior epigastric vessels in the right groin. It has no change on pressure or with Valsalva manoeuvre.

What is the most likely diagnosis?

(a) Recurrent direct inguinal hernia

(b) Recurrent indirect inguinal hernia

(c) Lymph node

(d) Lipoma

(e) Seroma

41. A 20-year-old runner presents with a history of right leg pain for 4 weeks. Radiography of the right leg shows a transverse cortical lucency and cortical thickening in the anterior cortex of the mid shaft of the tibia.

What is the most likely diagnosis?

(a) Stress fracture

(b) Nutrient artery foramen

(c) Osteomalacia

(d) Normal variant

(e) Hypertrophic pulmonary osteoarthropathy

42. An 18-year-old football player presents with right groin pain after a tackle. The radiograph shows avulsion of the lesser trochanter.

Which muscle is attached to the lesser trochanter?

(a) Sartorius

(b) Rectus femoris

(c) Iliopsoas

(d) Hamstrings

(e) Adductor longus

43. A 70-year-old man presents after falling down five stairs and sustaining injury to the neck. An open-mouth view shows increased space between the dens and medial border of lateral masses of C1. CT shows fracture of the anterior and posterior arch of the C1 vertebra.

What is the most likely diagnosis?

(a) Hangman's fracture
(b) Clay shoveller's fracture
(c) Jefferson fracture
(d) Extension teardrop fracture
(e) Flexion teardrop fracture

44. A 15-year-old boy presents with pain and swelling in the hands. Radiographs show periarticular osteopenia, loss of joint space at the metacarpophalangeal joints and widened bases in the proximal phalanges. A periosteal reaction is seen in the metacarpal bones.

What is the most likely diagnosis?

(a) Juvenile rheumatoid arthritis
(b) Psoriatic arthropathy
(c) Scleroderma
(d) Systemic lupus erythematosus
(e) Dermatomyositis

45. A 40-year-old immigrant from south Asia with a history of sexually transmitted disease treated 20 years ago presents with a painless, swollen right knee. Radiograph of the right knee shows collapse and fragmentation of the medial femoral condyle with subluxation of tibiofemoral joint. There is calcified debris in the knee and a large joint effusion. The bones show excessive sclerosis.

What is the most likely diagnosis?

(a) Diabetes
(b) Haemophilia
(c) Charcot's joint
(d) Calcium pyrophosphate deposition disease
(e) Osteoarthritis

46. A 42-year-old man in remission for lymphoma complains of bilateral hip pain. Coronal T1 images on MRI show geographical areas of abnormality in bilateral femoral heads, which are well demarcated from the normal bone by a thin rim of low signal on T1-weighted images.

What is the most likely diagnosis?

(a) Lymphoma recurrence
(b) Red bone marrow
(c) Avascular necrosis
(d) Osteomyelitis
(e) Stress fractures

47. A 70-year-old woman with a history of dysphagia presents with multiple swelling in the hands. Radiographs of the hands show widespread soft tissue calcification with terminal phalangeal resorption.

What is the most likely diagnosis?

(a) Systemic lupus erythematosus
(b) Scleroderma
(c) Dermatomyositis
(d) Psoriasis
(e) Calcium pyrophosphate deposition disease

48. A 60-year-old diabetic man with a 7-day-old compound fracture of the right tibia and fibula develops fever and septicaemia. Radiography of the leg shows a fracture of the mid shaft of tibia and fibula, along with extensive air in the soft tissues extending to the ankle and knee.

What is the most likely diagnosis?

(a) Air secondary to compound fracture
(b) Aerobic bacterial infection
(c) *Clostridium* infection
(d) *Staphylococcus* infection
(e) Beta-haemolytic streptococci

49. A 40-year-old man presents with progressive pain and swelling of the left knee joint. MRI shows extensive low-signal synovial masses around the right knee on T1, T2 and STIR sequences. There is marked degenerative joint disease as well.

What is the most likely diagnosis?

(a) Synovial chondromatosis
(b) Pigmented villonodular synovitis
(c) Synovial hypertrophy
(d) Lipoma arborescens
(e) Degenerative arthritis

50. A 14-year-old boy presents with persistent right hip pain after a recent injury. Radiographs confirm the diagnosis of slipped capital femoral epiphysis.

What is the Salter–Harris classification of this condition?

(a) Type I
(b) Type II
(c) Type III
(d) Type IV
(e) Type V

ANSWERS

1. **(b) Stress fracture**

   This is the most likely diagnosis as this is a very common site for stress fractures in the feet of runners, especially affecting the second and third metatarsals. Bone scan is almost 100% sensitive showing abnormal uptake within 6–72 hours of injury. MRI is also a very sensitive modality showing intermediate signal intensity on T1 and high signal on STIR and T2-weighted images.

2. **(b) Peripheral nerve sheath tumour**

   The location and direction of mobility along with typical MRI features clinch the diagnosis of peripheral nerve sheath tumour.

   Ganglion, lipoma and callous would not appear as hypervascular lesions. Liposarcoma can show increased vascularity but demonstrates heterogenous enhancement on MRI.

3. **(c) Intraosseous lipoma**

   This is an expansile, non-aggressive lesion usually seen in metaphyses. It may contain a focal area of dystrophic calcification within (secondary to fat necrosis). On MRI, the lesion returns fat signal on all sequences (high signal on T1 and T2, and low signal on STIR).

4. **(a) Unicameral bone cyst**

   This is usually asymptomatic unless fractured. The lesion usually is 2–3 cm in size, usually in the metaphysis, with its long axis parallel to the long axis of the bone. There may be endosteal scalloping of the bone and a 'fallen-fragment sign' (if fractured, centrally dislodged fracture fragment falls into a dependent position in the cyst).

5. **(d) Ewing's sarcoma with fracture**

   For a simple fracture with haematoma, this case has presented too early for a periosteal reaction. Neuroblastoma metastasis could be considered in a child less than 5 years old, and lymphoma should be considered in patients over 30 years age. Osteomyelitis could have been possible if there had been a previous history of localised pain, fever etc.

6. **(b) Renal osteodystrophy**

   Patients with renal osteodystrophy have extensive soft tissue calcifications, particularly in periarticular distribution. 'Superscan' appearance is also a feature.

7. **(a) Reflex sympathetic dystrophy**

This is commonly associated with trauma. The condition causes hyperhidrosis skin changes with excessive pitting oedema, sudomotor changes (hyperhidrosis and hypertrichosis), pain and patchy osteopenia. Three-phase bone scan shows increased blood flow, increased blood pool and increased periarticular uptake on delayed images.

8. **(c) Haemangioma**

Vertebral haemangiomas are visualised with fine or coarse vertical striations, commonly seen in vertebral bodies. CT shows a dotted appearance in a fatty matrix. On MRI, they present as lesions, returning high signal on T1 and T2 due to their high fat content.

Metastatic lesions are Intermediate signal on T1 and high on T2. Schmorl's node affects the end plates.

9. **(e) Osteoid osteoma**

This typically presents as a small lytic lesion with central mineralisation surrounded by reactive sclerotic area. On bone scans, the central nidus shows intense uptake surrounded by region of lesser activity (double density sign). MRI demonstrates bone oedema pattern and typically relieved with aspirin.

Stress fractures are transverse and linear. Ewing's sarcoma and infection must be considered if soft tissue involvement is seen on MRI.

10. **(b) Giant cell tumour**

Typical features on radiograph are a lytic, eccentric, expansile, subarticular lesion with 'soap bubble' appearance (fluid–fluid level on MRI).

Benign fibrous histiocytoma and telangiectatic osteosarcoma can also show fluid–fluid levels but are metaphyseal lesions not extending to the subarticular surface. A simple bone cyst is unilocular and situated away from the articular surface.

11. **(a) Gaucher's disease**

This is the commonest lipid storage disorder. Marrow infiltration leads to avascular necrosis in the femur, ankle and humerus. Patients have splenomegaly, anaemia and pancytopaenia. Loss of normal remodelling of the femur results in Erlenmeyer flask' deformity at the distal femur.

12. **(b) Pigmented villonodular synovitis**

This is a benign pathology affecting usually the knee joint. It shows no calcifications, osteoporosis or erosions (until late). MRI is diagnostic, the lesions returning low signal on all sequences due to iron (haemosiderin).

13. (c) Gouty arthritis

Periarticular erosions with sclerotic borders and overhanging margins with preserved articular surface are typical of gout.

Rheumatoid arthropathy has non-proliferative marginal erosions, symmetrical distribution and joint space narrowing. Psoriasis show progressive joint destruction with erosions. Erosive osteoarthritis is symmetrical with erosions are the articular surface Calcium pyrophosphate deposition disease is polyarticular, and shows chondrocalcinosis and joint-space narrowing.

14. (d) Hypertrophic osteoarthropathy

This is seen in multiple conditions (e.g. malignant tumours of the lung, some benign lesions, chronic chest infections). The condition manifests as cortical thickening and lamellar periosteal reaction in the diametaphyseal regions of the long bones. Bone scanning shows symmetrical uptake along the cortical margins of the diaphysis and metaphysis of tubular bones.

15. (b) Paget's disease

Asymmetrical cortical sclerosis and trabecular thickening is seen in Paget's disease.

Metastatic disease of the prostate is unlike to affect only a hemipelvis and does not directly cause acetabular protrusion. Fluorosis causes generalised sclerosis of the bones in the body

16. (e) Meniscal cyst

Meniscal cysts are very commonly associated with meniscal tears. MRI shows classic features of the cyst, related to the parameniscal structures. Lateral meniscal cysts tend to be smaller but are often more symptomatic than cysts in the medial counterparts.

17. (b) Maffucci's syndrome

This diagnosis is a combination of multiple enchondromatosis and soft tissue haemangiomas. Hand and foot involvement is common and severe. The soft tissue calcifications are phleboliths from haemangiomas.

In Ollier's disease, there is absence of haemangioma and phleboliths.

18. (b) Erosive osteoarthritis

Central articular erosion with a 'seagull' pattern, ankylosis and periarticular osteoporosis is typical of erosive osteoarthritis. This is seen in older women and is usually limited to hands, particularly affecting the proximal interphalangeal joints.

19. (b) Morton's neuroma

This is the typical ultrasound appearance of a Morton's neuroma. Treatment is conservative or surgical removal. On MRI the lesion appears as intermediate signal intensity on T1 and T2.

Bursitis is compressible on ultrasound probe pressure.

20. (b) Hypertrophic osteoarthropathy (HPOA) with rib fractures

On bone scan multiple areas of uptake in a linear pattern suggests traumatic injury to ribs. HPOA is characterised by bilateral symmetrical tracer uptake on bone scanning, involving the diaphyseal and metaphyseal regions of long bones. Characteristically a periosteal reaction is seen along the shafts of involved bones. This pattern of uptake is called a 'double-stripe' or 'parallel-track' sign and is characteristic of HPOA.

21. (d) Reflex sympathetic dystrophy

A history of trauma, periarticular uptake on bone scan and osteoporosis suggests reflex sympathetic dystrophy.

All other conditions are likely to affect both feet.

22. (b) Paget's disease

Paget's disease can be monostotic or polyostotic and demonstrates intense tracer uptake on bone scan. The area of uptake usually conforms well to the area of bone that is distorted or expanded. The most common bones involved are the pelvis, spine, skull, femur, scapula, tibia and humerus. Many patients are evaluated after finding increased serum alkaline phosphatase.

23. (c) Insufficiency fractures

Presence of bilateral sacral ala fractures with pubic fractures in this clinical context is virtually diagnostic of insufficiency fractures. Presence of marginal sclerosis at the fractures suggests chronic changes.

24. (c) Schatzker type 3

Type 1 is lateral condylar split, type 2 is lateral split with depression, type 3 is pure lateral depression, type 4 is medial condylar fracture and depression, type 5 is bicondylar fracture and type 6 is fracture extending to metadiaphysis.

25. (a) Iliopsoas muscle

This is attached to the lesser trochanter.

26. (b) Monteggia fracture dislocation

This involves a fracture of the proximal ulna shaft with dislocated radial head.

27. (a) Bone infarct

The radiographic and MRI appearances described are typical for a bone infarct. These are typically metaphyseal or diaphyseal in contrast to osteonecrosis. Bone scans may show increased uptake in acute stages where revascularisation has occurred.

28. (a) Spontaneous osteonecrosis of knee

Typical subchondral fracture in elderly patient after minor knee injury.

29. (e) Lipoma arborescens

This condition is seen most commonly in the suprapatellar pouch, with small to large frond-like masses arising from synovium. On MRI, the masses show characteristic signal of fat on all sequences. Saturation on STIR images is diagnostic.

30. (b) Plantar fibromatosis

This presents as nodular thickening in the plantar fascia. There can be single or multiple lesions. On MRI, the lesion is low signal on T1 and mild hyperintensity on T2, and the nodule enhances with gadolinium.

31. (d) Parosteal lipoma

These are benign tumours of adipose tissue which are intimately related to the periosteum. They often contain bony excrescences that may resemble osteochondroma but, unlike osteochondroma, they do not communicate with the medullary cavity of parent bone. MRI is diagnostic, confirming the juxtacortical benign nature of the fatty lesion and non-communication of the bony lesion with the medulla of the adjacent bone.

32. (a) Osteochondroma

The best diagnostic feature of osteochondroma is continuity of the bony cortex and medulla with the parent bone.

33. (b) Enchondroma

Radiographic features are typical and diagnostic. A bone infarct appears as a serpiginous area with sclerotic margins and no endosteal scalloping.

Chondrosarcoma shows periosteal reaction and an associated soft tissue mass.

34. **(b) Osteoblastoma**

    Also called giant osteoid osteoma when measuring > 2 cm.

    Osteoid osteoma are < 2 cm, have a predilection for the axial skeleton and usually respond to salicylates. Osteosarcomas show cortical destruction, mineralised matrix and soft tissue mass. Aneurysmal bone cysts show fluid–fluid levels and no matrix calcification.

35. **(b) Osteoma**

    The best diagnostic clue is the densely sclerotic, well-defined lesion attached to the parent bone. Latent lesions show no tracer uptake.

36. **(a) Anterior cruciate ligament**

    The anterior cruciate ligament is attached to the medial part of the tibial spine.

37. **(c) Avascular necrosis**

    Avascular necrosis of the femoral head is a complication after hip dislocation. It may be seen as a wedge-shaped or geographical area of subchondral ischemic focus in the weight-bearing area. On MRI, there is a hyperintense inner border parallel to a hypointense periphery.

38. **(a) Direct inguinal hernia**

    A direct inguinal hernia is seen medial to the inferior epigastric vessels whereas an indirect hernia is seen lateral to them.

39. **(b) Indirect inguinal hernia**

    An indirect inguinal hernia protrudes through the internal inguinal ring and extends along the inguinal canal parallel to its long axis.

40. **(d) Lipoma**

    The lesion has typical sonographic characteristics of a lipoma.

41. **(a) Stress fracture**

    This is commonly seen in runners and other athletes, in marching soldiers and in other patients in whom repetitive prolonged muscular action and stress are applied to a bone that is not accustomed to such action.

42. **(a) Iliopsoas**

    Iliopsoas is attached to the lesser trochanter.

43. (c) Jefferson fracture

Jefferson fracture involves the C1 vertebra. There is a comminuted fracture of the C1 ring, at least through two places. Plain radiography using an open-mouth view demonstrates lateral displacement of the lateral masses.

44. (a) Juvenile rheumatoid arthritis

The condition is usually seen in young people before the age of 16 years. In the hand, the metacarpophalangeal and interphalangeal joints are usually affected. Chronic synovitis causes enlargement of bones and epiphyses. Malalignment and subluxation are common. An important feature of juvenile arthritis is periosteal reaction affecting the metacarpal and phalangeal shafts.

45. (c) Charcot's joint

The radiographic features are those of Charcot's joint. Given the history of treated sexually transmitted disease, syphilis must be considered.

46. (c) Avascular necrosis

This appearance on MRI is typical of avascular necrosis.

47. (b) Scleroderma

Scleroderma is the cutaneous manifestation of progressive systemic sclerosis. This causes fibrosis and small vessel disease in several organs. In the hands, typically it causes terminal phalangeal resorption due to pressure atrophy, soft tissue calcification and occasionally intra-articular calcification.

48. (c) *Clostridium* infection

Gas in the soft tissues after compound fractures is a manifestation of infection. Gas gangrene after *Clostridium* infection is a classical example and causes extensive oedema, necrosis of tissues with gas production resulting in a severe toxic state.

Other gas-forming organisms include anaerobic bacteria, coliforms and Bacteroides.

49. (b) Pigmented villonodular synovitis

The MRI appearances described are typical of pigmented villonodular synovitis, showing low signal of abnormal synovium on all sequences.

50. (e) Type I Salter–Harris injury

Slipped capital femoral epiphysis is classified as a type I Salter–Harris injury because there is a slipped epiphysis due to the shearing force of an injury, separating the epiphysis from the metaphysis. There is no fracture of the metaphysis or the epiphysis itself.

Chapter 3

Gastrointestinal system

QUESTIONS

1. An 18-year-old woman who is 12 weeks pregnant has a routine ultrasound examination for non-specific abdominal pain. The scan demonstrates a 1.5 cm well-defined, hyperechoic, lobulated and homogenous lesion in the right lobe of the liver. Doppler ultrasound shows no significant signal within the lesion.

   The most likely cause is?

   (a) Metastasis
   (b) Haemangioma
   (c) Focal nodular hyperplasia
   (d) Hepatic adenoma
   (e) Focal fat deposition

2. A 65-year-old woman is admitted with abdominal pain. ERCP shows generalised dilated intrahepatic and extrahepatic ducts with multifocal strictures and small diverticulae formation.

   The most likely diagnosis is?

   (a) Primary sclerosing cholangitis
   (b) Choledochocoele
   (c) Caroli's syndrome
   (d) Cholangiocarcinoma
   (e) Primary biliary cirrhosis

3. A 35-year-old woman with mucocutaneous pigmentation on the hands and feet and in a circumoral distribution presents with cramping abdominal pain. She is found to have iron deficiency anaemia. Plain radiography of the abdomen suggested small bowel obstruction. Contrast-enhanced CT demonstrates jejunal intussusception.

    The most likely diagnosis is?

    (a) Familial adenomatous polyposis
    (b) Peutz–Jeghers syndrome
    (c) Leiomyoma small bowel
    (d) Small bowel carcinoma
    (e) Melanoma with bowel metastases.

4. A 40-year-old woman who takes contraceptive pills is admitted with right upper quadrant pain and menorrhagia. She had a skin lesion excised by a dermatologist 5 years previously. CT shows multiple enhancing lesions in the liver. MRI demonstrates multiple homogenous hepatic lesions with increased signal intensity on T1 images.

    The most likely diagnosis is?

    (a) Bronchogenic carcinoma with hepatic metastases
    (b) Melanoma metastases
    (c) Colorectal metastases
    (d) Multiple haemangiomas
    (e) Hepatic adenomas

5. A 60-year-old heavy goods vehicle driver presents with abdominal pain. Ultrasound shows a 5 cm area of increased echogenicity adjacent to the gallbladder. T1 in-phase gradient-echo MRIs show the lesion isointense to the liver parenchyma while the T1 out-of-phase images demonstrate a focal area of signal loss in the region.

    The most likely diagnosis is?

    (a) Focal nodular hyperplasia
    (b) Focal hepatic steatosis.
    (c) Haemangioma
    (d) Metastatic deposit from melanoma
    (e) Focal fatty sparing

6. A 35-year-old man with history of multiple scalp lesions and dental caries presents with abdominal pain and vomiting. CT of the abdomen shows extensive colonic lesions and a duodenal mass causing partial obstruction.

    The most likely diagnosis is?

    (a) Familial adenomatous polyposis
    (b) Lymphoma
    (c) Inflammatory polyps
    (d) Ulcerative colitis
    (e) Whipple's disease

7. To differentiate between a renal cell carcinoma which has spread into the perinephric fat and an angiomyolipoma with haemorrhage, the best diagnostic modality would be?

    (a) Ultrasound
    (b) CT scan
    (c) MRI
    (d) Angiogram
    (e) Cannot be differentiated

8. A 50-year-old primary school teacher presents with history of recurrent episodes of loss of consciousness. CT scan of the abdomen shows a enhancing mass in the pancreas.

    The most likely diagnosis is?

    (a) Pancreatic carcinoma
    (b) Gastrinoma
    (c) Lymphoma
    (d) Insulinoma
    (e) Adrenocorticotrophic hormone-producing tumour

9. Which of the following investigations is the most sensitive test for localisation of Islet cell tumours?

    (a) Transhepatic portal venous sampling (TPVS)
    (b) Contrast enhanced MRI
    (c) Endoscopic ultrasound
    (d) Selective arteriography
    (e) Arterial stimulation and venous sampling (ASVS)

10. A patient with history of underlying heart condition was diagnosed with a liver lesion.

Which of the following is a contraindication for ultrasound-guided liver biopsy?

(a) HIV positive patient

(b) INR 1.5

(c) Suspected metastasis

(d) Suspected haemangioma

(e) Obesity

11. A 60-year-old man was admitted with intermittent abdominal pain. CT scan shows an ill-defined soft tissue mass in the bowel mesentery, with extensive calcification within. Strands of soft tissue are seen radiating into the surrounding fatty mesentery. The adjacent bowel loops show retraction. MRI shows low signal on T1 and T2 images.

The most likely diagnosis is?

(a) Carcinoid syndrome

(b) Fibrosing mesenteritis

(c) Mesenteric panniculitis

(d) Desmoid tumour

(e) Old tuberculosis

12. A 40-year-old man presented with left lower abdominal pain. A CT scan demonstrates a 2 cm fat density lesion surrounded by a hyperdense rim and inflammatory fat stranding abutting the sigmoid colon although no wall thickening or sigmoid diverticulosis was seen.

The most likely diagnosis is?

(a) Appendicitis

(b) Epiploic appendagitis

(c) Diverticulitis

(d) Mesenteric panniculitis

(e) Omental infarction

13. A 40-year-old white man with insulin-dependent diabetes and hyperpigmentation presents with renal colic. A non-contrast CT scan is performed which shows generalised increase in liver attenuation. Later, MRI shows homogenous signal loss in the liver on T2.

The most likely cause of liver appearances is?

(a) Diffuse fatty liver
(b) Biliary cirrhosis
(c) Thorotrast injection previously
(d) Haemochromatosis
(e) Normal variant

14. A 30-year-old man presents with weight loss and diarrhoea. There is family history of father having total colectomy at age of 21 years. On colonoscopy the patient is found to have hundreds of polyps in the colon. CT shows a enhancing mass in the second part of duodenum.

The most likely diagnosis is?

(a) Juvenile polyposis
(b) Familial adenomatous polyposis
(c) Metaplastic polyposis
(d) Peutz–Jeghers syndrome
(e) Turcot's syndrome

15. A 35-year-old mother on oral contraceptives presents with vague abdominal pain. Ultrasound was normal. MRI demonstrates a 3 cm, well-defined lesion in the right lobe of liver that is homogenous except for a central scar. The lesion returns low signal on T1 and slightly higher signal on T2 as compared with liver. With gadolinium, the lesion shows enhancement in arterial phase and is isointense in portovenous phase. The central scar shows late and prolonged enhancement.

The most likely diagnosis is?

(a) Hepatic adenoma
(b) Hepatocellular carcinoma
(c) Giant cavernous haemangioma
(d) Focal nodular hyperplasia
(e) Metastasis

16. A 50-year-old woman presents with symptoms of acute cholecystitis. Ultrasound shows an incidental 3 cm hyperechoic lesion in the spleen. Contrast-enhanced CT shows that the lesion enhances poorly. On MRI, the lesion is isointense to spleen on T1 and bright on T2. With gadolinium, there is a centripetal pattern enhancement.

    The most likely diagnosis is?

    (a) Haemangioma
    (b) Acute haematoma
    (c) Simple cyst
    (d) Cystic metastasis
    (e) Lymphangioma

17. A 60-year-old man with history of aortic valve replacement presents with bleeding per rectum. Colonoscopy is normal. On arteriography, a cluster of vessels are seen on the antimesenteric border of the ascending colon, with early opacification of the ileocolic vein.

    The most likely diagnosis is?

    (a) Occult carcinoma
    (b) Angiodysplasia
    (c) Gastrointestinal stromal tumour
    (d) Portal hypertension
    (e) Diverticulitis

18. A 48-year-old woman presents with history of upper abdominal pain, weight loss and bilateral ankle oedema. CT abdomen shows thickened gastric wall with prominent mucosal folds affecting the upper part of the stomach and greater curvature, while the antrum, pylorus and rest of the bowel appear normal.

    The most likely diagnosis is?

    (a) Crohn's disease
    (b) Gastric carcinoma
    (c) Lymphoma
    (d) Ménétrier's disease
    (e) Eosinophilic gastritis

19. A 45-year-old man presents with acute-onset abdominal pain. Imaging confirms the diagnosis of intussusception.

    Which of the following is the most likely cause?

    (a) Meckel's diverticulum
    (b) Aberrant pancreas
    (c) Chronic tuberculosis ulcer
    (d) Scleroderma
    (e) Idiopathic

20. A 40-year-old patient presents with symptoms of recurrent asthma, heart failure and non-specific abdominal pain after meals and alcohol. CT shows a mass with desmoplastic reaction in the terminal ileum. The liver shows multiple lesions enhancing in the arterial phase.

    The most likely diagnosis is?

    (a) Carcinoid tumour of terminal ileum
    (b) Carcinoma of the terminal ileum with liver metastases
    (c) Lymphoma
    (d) Fibrosing mesenteritis
    (e) Carcinoid syndrome

21. A 6-year-old girl presents with gradually increasing abdominal mass. Plain radiography shows a soft tissue mass displacing the bowel loops, with small calcifications. Ultrasound reveals a 10 cm, thin walled, cystic lesion in the mid abdomen, with multiple internal septations and small internal echoes.

    The most likely diagnosis is?

    (a) Duplication cyst
    (b) Mesenteric cyst
    (c) Neuroblastoma
    (d) Ovarian cyst
    (e) Lymphoma

22. A 60-year-old diabetic man presents with fever, abdominal pain and jaundice. Ultrasound shows a 4 cm, well-defined, hypoechoic lesion with debris in the right lobe. CT shows a ill-defined, low-attenuating lesion with enhancing margins.

    The most likely diagnosis is?

    (a) Simple liver cyst
    (b) Haemangioma
    (c) Pyogenic liver abscess
    (d) Amoebic liver abscess
    (e) Hydatid cyst

23. An 18-year-old involved in a road traffic accident presents at the Accident & Emergency Department with abdominal pain. CT shows fat stranding in the small bowel mesentery. There is small amount of fluid between small bowel folds, with a Hounsfield unit of 75.

    The most likely diagnosis is?

    (a) Mesenteric haematoma
    (b) Splenic rupture
    (c) Liver laceration
    (d) Bowel perforation
    (e) Normal free fluid

24. A 50-year-old woman is admitted with right upper quadrant pain. Ultrasound shows a large gallstone within the lumen. The wall of the gallbladder is thickened and there are multiple echogenic intramural foci with 'comet tail' reverberation artefacts.

    The most likely cause of the reverberation artefacts is?

    (a) Adenomyomatosis
    (b) Gallbladder wall calcification
    (c) Gallbladder carcinoma in situ
    (d) Gallbladder papilloma
    (e) Gangrenous cholecystitis

25. A 60-year-old diabetic man presents with pain in the right upper quadrant. A plain abdominal radiographs show multiple calcified gallstones and an air fluid level in the gallbladder. Ultrasound shows air in the gallbladder wall.

The most likely diagnosis is?

(a) Enteric fistula
(b) Incompetent sphincter of Oddi
(c) Emphysematous cholecystitis
(d) Xanthogranulomatous cholecystitis
(e) Adenomyomatosis

26. A 60-year-old man presents with abdominal pain. Enteroclysis shows a contrast filling abnormality in the concavity of the second part of the duodenum. Contrast-enhanced CT shows two 'duodenal lumina'. The medial lumen contains an air-fluid level and causes medial displacement of the pancreatic head.

The most likely diagnosis is?

(a) Duodenal duplication cyst
(b) Duodenal diverticulum
(c) Pancreatic pseudocyst
(d) Pancreatic tumour
(e) Necrotic duodenal carcinoma

27. A 65-year-old woman presents with non-specific abdominal discomfort. Contrast-enhanced abdominal shows a homogenous, extraluminal mass with heterogeneous enhancement and a low attenuation centre arising from the greater curvature of stomach. No lymphadenopathy is seen. A subsequent PET scan shows markedly increased glucose uptake by the lesion.

What is the most likely diagnosis?

(a) Carcinoma of the stomach
(b) Gastrointestinal stromal tumour
(c) Lymphoma
(d) Carcinoid
(e) Metastases

28. A 60-year-old man presents with constipation and painful defecation. CT shows a non-enhancing, well-defined, lobulated, and homogenous, low-attenuation lesion in the retrorectal space. The lesion shows thin peripheral calcification. On MRI, the lesion returns intermediate signal on T1 with areas of high signal within and high signal on T2 with septae.

What is the most likely diagnosis?

(a) Enteric cyst
(b) Dermoid cyst
(c) Sacrococcygeal teratoma
(d) Anal duct cyst
(e) Rectal leiomyosarcoma

29. A 40-year-old man presents with a 4-week history of right iliac fossa pain. Ultrasound shows a tubular fluid filed lesion in the right lower abdomen. CT shows a homogenous prominent appendix of high attenuation (30 Hounsfield units). No inflammatory change, calcifications, lymph nodes or free fluid are seen.

The most likely diagnosis is?

(a) Normal appendix
(b) Lymphoma of the appendix
(c) Mucocoele of the appendix
(d) Carcinoma of the appendix
(e) Carcinoid of the appendix

30. A chronic alcoholic presents with gradually increasing abdominal distension and pedal oedema. Ultrasound shows a small nodular liver and ascites, and Doppler shows absence of blood flow in the left and middle hepatic veins.

What is the most likely cause of absence of blood flow in hepatic veins?

(a) Budd–Chiari syndrome
(b) Cirrhosis of the liver
(c) Hepatoma
(d) Cavernous transformation of the portal vein
(e) None of the above

31. A 40-year-old patient with acute myeloid leukaemia on chemotherapy presents with acute-onset pain in the right lower abdomen and diarrhoea. CT shows circumferential thickening of the caecal wall and mild surrounding inflammatory changes in the mesenteric fat.

    What is the most likely diagnosis?

    (a) Epiploic appendagitis
    (b) Typhlitis
    (c) Ulcerative colitis
    (d) Crohn's disease
    (e) Ischaemic colitis

32. A 50-year-old woman with a history of bleeding per rectum presents for a barium enema. The examination shows multiple worm-like projections attached by their bases to the sigmoid colon.

    The most likely diagnosis is?

    (a) Postinflammatory polyps
    (b) Juvenile polyps
    (c) Familial adenomatous polyposis
    (d) Faecal residue
    (e) Colonic ulceration

33. A 60-year-old alcoholic presents with gradual distension of abdomen. He gives a history of surgically treated complicated appendicitis. Ultrasound shows extensive thin-walled cystic masses in the abdomen.

    The most likely diagnosis is?

    (a) Ascites
    (b) Peritoneal metastases
    (c) Pseudomyxoma peritonei
    (d) Pancreatic pseudocyst
    (e) Pyogenic peritonitis

34. A 30-year-old man presents with history of intermittent abdominal pain for 1 month. Serum lipase and amylase were markedly raised. CT shows pancreatitis with multiple calcifications in the pancreas and focal fatty change adjacent to the falciform ligament. MRI shows that the common bile duct and the ventral pancreatic duct drain into the major papilla, and the dorsal pancreatic duct drains the minor papilla.

The most likely diagnosis is?

(a) Annular pancreas
(b) Pancreas divisum
(c) Normal pancreas
(d) Aberrant common bile duct
(e) Ectopic pancreas

35. A 27-year-old Asian man presents with fever and abdominal pain. CT shows hepatosplenomegaly with multiple cervical, mediastinal and para-aortic lymph nodes.

The most likely diagnosis is?

(a) Non-Hodgkin's lymphoma
(b) Lymphoma
(c) Diffuse metastatic disease
(d) Sarcoidosis
(e) Malaria

36. A 70-year-old man with history of CVA and coronary artery bypass grafting presents with bloody diarrhoea, abdominal pain and vomiting. Blood gases show severe metabolic acidosis. CT abdomen shows focal area of thickened sigmoid flexure with pericolic stranding and normal right colon.

The most likely diagnosis is?

(a) Ulcerative colitis
(b) Ischaemic colitis
(c) Infection
(d) Crohn's disease
(e) Pseudomembranous colitis

37. A 35-year-old previously fit man presents with abdominal pain and a lump in right lower abdomen. CT shows a hernia just lateral to the right rectus muscle with an obstructed loop of small bowel.

What is the likely diagnosis?

(a) Ventral hernia
(b) Spigelian hernia
(c) Umbilical hernia
(d) Hernia through a laparoscopic port
(e) Inguinal hernia

38. A 45-year-old man with a history of laparotomy presents with palpable hard lump in the abdominal wall. CT shows a soft tissue mass with ill-defined margins in the rectus muscle showing mild contrast enhancement. On MRI, the lesion returns low signal on T1 and T2.

What is the most likely diagnosis?

(a) Desmoid
(b) Metastasis
(c) Haematoma
(d) Seroma
(e) Lymphoma

39. A 50-year-old woman with a history of complicated appendix surgery in the past presents with abdominal pain and distension. CT shows diffuse cystic abnormalities in the abdomen pushing the bowel loops centrally, filling the lesser sac with scalloping of the hepatic and splenic margins.

What is the most likely diagnosis?

(a) Peritoneal metastases
(b) Peritoneal sarcomatosis
(c) Pseudomyxoma peritonei
(d) TB peritonitis
(e) Bacterial peritonitis

40. A 47-year-old diabetic man with recent renal transplant, presents with dysphagia. Double-contrast barium swallow shows longitudinally oriented filling defects in the upper and mid oesophagus. CT shows circumferential thickening of the upper half of oesophagus.

What is the most likely diagnosis?

(a) Reflux oesophagitis
(b) Viral oesophagitis
(c) *Candida* oesophagitis
(d) Oesophageal varices
(e) Carcinoma

41. A 21-year-old man presents with dysphagia and weight loss. Barium swallow shows absence of a primary peristaltic wave and a dilated and tortuous oesophagus with a smooth, tapered narrowing at the oesophago-gastric junction.

What is the most likely diagnosis?

(a) Oesophageal carcinoma
(b) Achalasia of the oesophagus
(c) Gastric carcinoma
(d) Peptic stricture
(e) Diffuse oesophageal spasm

42. A 28-year-old man smelling of alcohol presented to the casualty department with chest pain and vomiting. The chest radiograph shows pneumomediastinum, surgical emphysema and left hydropneumothorax.

What is the most likely diagnosis?

(a) Mallory–Weiss syndrome
(b) Boerhaave syndrome
(c) Spontaneous pneumothorax
(d) Post traumatic
(e) None of the above

43. A 70-year-old man presents with acute onset pain and distension of the abdomen. Abdominal radiograph shows a dilated, inverted 'U' shaped sigmoid colon. No gas is seen in the rectum. Single-contrast barium enema shows a smooth, curved tapering of the barium column like a hooked beak at the distal colon.

    What is the most likely diagnosis?

    (a) Sigmoid volvulus
    (b) Caecal volvulus
    (c) Acute ileus
    (d) Functional megacolon
    (e) Toxic megacolon

44. A 40-year-old man with history of lymphoma presents with recurrent haematemesis. The chest radiograph shows mediastinal widening. Mucosal relief views on barium study show tortuous, serpiginous, longitudinal radiolucent filling defects in the upper oesophagus. Endoscopic ultrasound shows multiple anechoic spaces in the submucosal region with thin walls.

    What is the most likely diagnosis of the appearance in barium study?

    (a) Oesophagitis ulceration
    (b) Superior vena cava obstruction with downhill varices
    (c) *Candida* oesophagitis
    (d) Oesophageal pseudodiverticulosis
    (e) Primary oesophageal lymphoma

45. A 50-year-old obese woman presents with abdominal pain and abnormal liver function tests. MRI shows diffuse low signal intensity of the liver on T1 out-of-phase gradient echo images.

    What is the most likely diagnosis?

    (a) Diffuse lymphoma
    (b) Fatty liver
    (c) Acute hepatitis
    (d) Primary biliary cirrhosis
    (e) Hepatic sarcoidosis

46. A 30-year-old man presents with non-specific epigastric pain. Ultrasound shows a 2 cm anechoic lesion in segment 2 of the liver. This has smooth margins with no-detectable walls, no septations or mural nodules are seen. On contrast-enhanced CT the lesion has a Hounsfield unit of 10.

What is the most likely diagnosis?

(a) Necrotic metastases
(b) Haemangioma
(c) Simple hepatic cyst
(d) Pyogenic abscess
(e) Hydatid cyst

47. A 37-year-old woman presents with epigastric pain and weight loss. Barium meal shows multiple small barium collections with surrounding lucent halos in the distal body and antrum of stomach.

The most likely diagnosis is?

(a) Gastric metastases
(b) Gastric varices
(c) Erosive gastritis
(d) Gastric polyps
(e) Menetrier disease

48. A 70-year-old man with history of history of alcoholism, presents with progressive dysphagia. Barium studies of the upper gastrointestinal tract show irregular narrowing of the oesophagus just above the gastro-oesophageal junction, with abrupt transition to normal mucosa proximally.

What is the most likely diagnosis?

(a) Ulcerating carcinoma of the oesophagus
(b) Barrett's oesophagus
(c) Schatzki rings
(d) Oesophageal polyps
(e) Achalasia of oesophagus

49. A 70-year-old woman under investigation for anaemia and upper abdominal pain has barium study of the upper gastrointestinal tract, which shows a featureless tubular narrow stomach. The area gastricae are absent.

What is the most likely diagnosis?

(a) *Helicobacter pylori* gastritis
(b) Crohn's disease
(c) Atrophic gastritis
(d) Ménétrier's disease
(e) Zollinger–Ellison syndrome

50. A 60-year-old woman presents with history of acid reflux disease and chronic cough. The chest radiograph shows a 5 cm retrocardiac shadow in the midline with an air–fluid level.

What is the most likely diagnosis?

(a) Bronchogenic cyst
(b) Lung abscess
(c) Hiatus hernia
(d) Bronchogenic carcinoma
(e) Left lower lobe collapse

ANSWERS

1. **(b) Haemangioma**

    This is the commonest lesion seen with described appearance on ultrasound.

    Metastasis is also less likely given the age and features. Focal fatty deposition usually has angular margins and a 'geographic appearance' on ultrasound. Focal nodular hyperplasia has similar reflectivity to liver on ultrasound and may show mass effect. A Doppler signal can often be seen in the lesion.

2. **(a) Primary sclerosing cholangitis**

    These features are typically diagnostic of primary sclerosing cholangitis.

    Caroli's disease is rare condition which manifests in childhood, adolescents and into the third decade. Appearances can be similar to primary sclerosing cholangitis. Choledochocoele is seen in young adults: there is a sac-like dilatation of the intramural segment of the common bile duct which prolapses into the duodenum; there are scattered dilated intrahepatic ducts with no apparent connection to main bile ducts. Caudate lobe hypertrophy is seen in primary biliary cirrhosis. Cholangiocarcinoma may be seen as mass lesion with focal duct dilatation; no generalised strictures and diverticulae are seen.

3. **(b) Peutz–Jeghers syndrome**

    The syndrome presents with mucocutaneous pigmentation and gastrointestinal polyposis. Small bowel polyps may cause intussusception and anaemia.

    Other causes can have bowel lesions causing intussusception but do not show mucocutaneous lesions.

4. **(b) Malignant melanoma with hepatic metastases**

    Melanoma metastases show increased signal on T1 because of the paramagnetic effects of melanin itself. Most liver metastases show low signal on non-contrast T1 images unless there is intralesional haemorrhage, when they can be seen as heterogenous lesions.

5. **(b) Focal hepatic steatosis**

    Focal fatty infiltration is typically diagnosed with in-phase and out-of-phase MRI, where the area involved demonstrates signal loss in out-of-phase imaging. This can be due to many causes including diabetes, alcoholism and obesity. Common locations include tip of segment 4, along the ligament teres and adjacent to the gallbladder. On MRI, this feature is not seen in any of the other conditions listed.

6. **(a) Familial adenomatous polyposis**

    A combination of extensive colonic polyposis with extracolonic features such as osteoma of the skull and mandible, epidermoid cysts, abnormal dentition and desmoid tumours is called Gardner's syndrome and is now included as a part of the spectrum of familial adenomatous polyposis.

7. **(b) CT scan**

    Demonstration of fat within the mass will point to a diagnosis of angiomyolipoma.

8. **(d) Insulinoma**

    This is the most common functional islet cell tumour. It is characterised by the Whipple's triad of starvation, hypoglycaemia and relief with glucose. Patients can lose consciousness secondary to hypoglycaemia. The lesion enhances with contrast and has no predilection for any part of pancreas. On MRI, the tumour returns low signal on T1 and high on T2 images.

9. **(e) Arterial stimulation and venous sampling**

    This involves selective pancreatic arterial injection of a secretogogue and the hepatic venous flow is sampled. Lesions not seen on cross section imaging can be detected. The sensitivity of ASVS is same as TPVS for insulinoma but better for gastrinoma.

10. **(d) Suspected haemangioma**

    Other options are not contraindications for biopsy.

11. **(b) Fibrosing mesenteritis**

    This is the classical appearance for fibrosing mesenteritis.

12. **(b) Epiploic appendagitis**

    The typical appearance of this is a 2–4 cm fatty lesion surrounded by a rim of tissue and inflammatory change next to colon.

    An important differential is acute diverticulitis, which commonly has a background of diverticulosis and colonic wall thickening.

13. **(d) Haemochromatosis**

    In haemochromatosis there is excess deposition of iron in the liver resulting in increased density of the liver on CT and loss of T2 signal due to the paramagnetic effects of iron. This also causes skin pigmentation, diabetes and arthralgia.

14. (b) Familial adenomatous polyposis

By definition, hundreds of polyps have to be present for this diagnosis. It is an autosomal dominant condition and the polyps present around puberty. Almost all patients have duodenal adenomas, with a 5% risk of conversion to periampullary carcinoma.

Juvenile polyposis is rare and presents in infancy. Multiple metaplastic polyps are very rare. Peutz–Jeghers syndrome shows few colonic polyps, and most are seen in the small bowel. Turcot's syndrome is a rare association between colonic carcinoma and medulloblastoma.

15. (d) Focal nodular hyperplasia.

These are the typical features of focal nodular hyperplasia as seen on MRI.

Adenoma is heterogenous on all sequences and can be indistinguishable from hepatocellular carcinoma due to haemorrhage and necrosis. Haemangioma shows peripheral nodular enhancement with centripetal filling. Metastases are commonly heterogenous

16. (a) Haemangioma

Theses are typical radiological features of a splenic haemangioma.

A simple splenic cyst shows low signal on T1, high T2 and has no gadolinium enhancement. Lymphangioma behaves on MRI like simple cysts.

17. (b) Angiodysplasia

Angiodysplasia is associated with aortic stenosis and commonly found in the ascending colon. This is seen at the antimesenteric border. On angiography, there is cluster of vessels seen on arterial phase with early filling of the draining vessel. These can be small lesions and may be missed on colonoscopy.

18. (d) Ménétrier's disease

This is characterised by hypertrophy of gastric folds affecting the greater curvature while usually sparing the antrum, hypoproteinemia (causing ankle oedema) and hypochlorhydria.

Lymphoma involves any part of stomach and antrum. Eosinophilic gastritis often affects the antrum and the proximal small bowel. Crohn's disease shows multiple aphthous ulcers and commonly affects antrum and pylorus. It usually affects the terminal ileum as well.

19. (e) Idiopathic

Twenty per cent of all adult intussusceptions are idiopathic. The rest of the given causes are rare.

20. (e) Carcinoid syndrome

Carcinoid tumours most commonly arise from the small bowel or appendix. Liver metastases may result in carcinoid syndrome presenting with symptoms after food and alcohol.

21. (b) Mesenteric cyst

Mesenteric cysts are rare and are found in the mesentery and omentum. They are true congenital abnormalities and arise due to sequestration of mesenteric lymphatics. Imaging features are typical as given in this case history. CT scan defines the anatomic margins of the cyst but septations are poorly seen on CT. MRI features vary according to the contents of the cyst.

22. (c) Pyogenic liver abscess

A history of fever with the described imaging features is suggestive of this diagnosis.

Haemangioma is hyperechoic on ultrasound and shows centripetal filling with contrast. Amoebic abscess are uncommon in the UK and may show septations with nodular walls. On ultrasound and CT a hydatid cyst shows septations, daughter cysts, debris and calcifications. A simple liver cyst has no debris and shows no marginal enhancement.

23. (a) Mesenteric haematoma

Given the history of road traffic accident, high attenuating fluid between the bowel loops is likely to represent mesenteric injury.

24. (a) Adenomyomatosis

There is an underlying increase in the number and height of mucosal folds in the gallbladder. This frequently exists with cholelithiasis. Cholesterol crystals precipitate in the bile and are trapped in Rokitansky–Aschoff sinuses, which gives the typical 'comet tail' reverberation artefacts on ultrasound.

25. (c) Emphysematous cholecystitis

This is a result of ischaemia of the gallbladder wall and infection with gas-producing organisms. It is common in patients who have diabetes and is associated with gallstones. Intramural gas and intraluminal gas is highly suggestive of this diagnosis.

26. (b) Duodenal diverticulum

The most frequent location of a duodenal diverticulum is along the medial wall of the second or third part of the duodenum. Most patients are asymptomatic, however some may present with diverticulitis. Barium examination may show the classic 'windsock' deformity, with the contras-filled diverticulum seen to project into the true lumen or contrast-filled duodenum projecting medially into the 'C' of the duodenum.

Duodenal duplication cysts do not communicate with the true lumen of duodenum.

27. (b) Gastrointestinal stromal tumour

This is the likely diagnosis given the CT appearances. It presents as predominantly extraluminal masses with heterogeneously enhancing margins and a necrotic centre. Lymph node enlargement is not a feature.

Carcinomas show more vigorous local infiltration. Metastases from bowel are usually multiple and often present with a history of known primary malignancy. Lymphomas cause circumferential thickening with homogenous enhancement and lymph nodes. Carcinoids are mainly seen around terminal ileum and produce a desmoplastic reaction.

28. (a) Enteric cyst

Enteric cyst may be septated and filled with mucoid contents which return high signal on T1 images. On CT they have the characteristic features as in the case.

Dermoid cysts contain skin appendages and commonly contain fat. Sacrococcygeal teratomas are usually seen in paediatric age group. On CT and MRI, they appear as heterogeneously enhancing lesions with both cystic and solid components.

29. (a) Mucocoele of the appendix

A mucocoele is a chronic cystic dilatation of the appendiceal lumen caused by mucin collection. On ultrasound it is anechoic or hypoechoic, depending on the composition of mucous. On CT the lesion is homogenous and cystic. On MRI a mucocoele is hyperintense on T2 and hypo-isointense on T1.

30. (a) Budd–Chiari syndrome

This is caused by obstruction of one or more hepatic veins or the inferior vena cava. If the hepatic veins are seen on the grey scale but no flow is identified and reversed flow is not seen, Budd–Chiari syndrome is likely. There are numerous causes for Budd–Chiari syndrome, but most commonly it is idiopathic.

31. **(b) Typhlitis**

Given the history of acute myeloid leukaemia with chemotherapy, this is the most likely diagnosis.

32. **(a) Postinflammatory polyps**

Filiform polyps adhering to the colon by their bases are typical of postinflammatory polyps, which can be seen in ulcerative colitis.

33. **(c) Pseudomyxoma peritonei**

This is due to intraperitoneal rupture of an appendiceal or ovarian mucinous adenoma. The ascites is typically septated and there are several thin-walled cystic masses throughout the abdominal cavity.

34. **(b) Pancreas divisum**

This is the most common anatomical variant of the pancreas and is due to failure of fusion of the ventral and dorsal pancreatic buds. As a result, the main dorsal pancreatic duct drains through the minor papilla while the ventral pancreatic duct with the common bile duct drains through the major papilla.

35. **(a) Non-Hodgkin's lymphoma**

Hodgkin's lymphoma may but uncommonly cause hepatosplenomegaly.

36. **(b) Ischaemic colitis**

Ischaemic colitis is usually due to indolent non-occlusive atherosclerosis in the elderly. Colonic wall thickening in a watershed area suggests ischaemia as the aetiology. Risk factors include cardiovascular disease, diabetes, vasculitis, etc. On CT, there is colonic wall thickening (> 5 mm), in a watershed distribution. The colon wall may appear non-enhancing compared with normal colon or it may appear dense due to haemorrhage. Pneumatosis coli, portal vein gas and perforation may be found.

37. **(b) Spigelian hernia**

This is seen through weakness in the spigelian aponeurosis, which lies between the linea semilunaris laterally and the rectus muscle medially.

Ventral hernia is usually midline, through the linea alba.

38. **(a) Desmoid**

The lesion is fibrous tissue returning low signal on T1 and T2 sequences. There is usually a history of abdominal surgery and the lesions are 'rock hard'.

Other differentials are unlikely given the imaging characteristics.

39. (c) Pseudomyxoma peritonei

The hint is the history of complicated appendix surgery. Pseudomyxoma peritonei is secondary to ruptured adenocarcinoma appendix, causing diffuse intraperitoneal accumulation of gelatinous ascites. The diagnostic CT features are a liver and spleen that have scalloped margins, along with low-attenuation masses that push the bowels centrally.

Peritoneal sarcomatosis cause haemorrhagic masses with solid and cystic components.

40. (c) *Candida* oesophagitis

This is seen in immunocompromised patients and is caused by Candida species. It spares the lower oesophagus and typically shows longitudinally oriented filling defects on double-contrast barium swallow.

Reflux usually extends proximally from gastro-oesophageal junction with ulcers in distal oesophagus. Viral oesophagitis (due to herpes virus or cytomegalovirus) usually shows multiple discrete ulcers. Cytomegalovirus may show giant ulcers (> 1 cm). Varices show serpiginous longitudinal defects, best seen on mucosal relief views.

41. (b) Achalasia of the oesophagus

This is a primary motility disorder which is secondary to failure of organised peristalsis and relaxation at the oesophago-gastric junction. A 'bird beak' or 'rat tail' appearance of distal oesophagus is typical on a barium swallow study.

Oesophageal and gastric carcinoma show mucosal irregularity, shouldering and mass effect. Peptic strictures are commonly associated with a hiatus hernia and show small mucosal ulcers. Diffuse oesophageal spasm is seen as a 'cork screw' appearance on barium study.

42. (b) Boerhaave syndrome

This is characterised by spontaneous distal oesophageal perforation following vomiting or violent straining. The tear usually is seen at the left lateral wall of distal oesophagus just above the oesophago-gastric junction. Diagnosis is made by demonstrating leak of extraluminal air and contrast around oesophagus. A perforated Mallory–Weiss tear is a Boerhaave syndrome.

43. (a) Sigmoid volvulus

This usually occurs when the sigmoid loop twists around the mesenteric axis. There are many radiological signs on plain radiographs and on single contrast barium enema a typical 'bird of prey' sign is seen.

44. (b) Downhill oesophageal varices secondary to superior vena cava obstruction

Mucosal relief views are suggestive of oesophageal varices secondary to superior vena cava obstruction by enlarged mediastinal nodes. Downhill varices usually involve upper half of the oesophagus while the uphill varices involve the lower half.

45. (b) Fatty liver

Ultrasound shows diffuse increased liver echogenicity, on CT the liver shows reduced attenuation as compared to the spleen, and on MRI a fatty liver returns low signal on T1 out-of-phase gradient echo images while in-phase images show increased signal intensity of liver compared with spleen.

46. (c) Simple hepatic cyst

These features are typical of a simple cyst. Patients are generally asymptomatic and the cysts are usually an incidental finding. Haemorrhage or infection in the cysts may cause pain.

47. (c) Erosive gastritis

The condition is characterised by aphthous ulcers seen as multiple small mucosal mounds, each having a central and superficial erosion (not penetrating the muscularis), in the antrum and body of stomach. The central erosion collects barium, with the mucosal mounds representing surrounding lucencies.

48. (a) Ulcerating carcinoma of the oesophagus

In patients with risk factors and irregular stricture in the oesophagus, carcinoma should be considered as first diagnosis and direct visualisation with histopathology is recommended.

49. (c) Atrophic gastritis

In elderly patients, this is associated with pernicious anaemia. The condition is characterised by loss of parietal cells leading to achlorhydria and atrophy of mucosa and mucosal glands. Radiographic findings as described in the case history are typical of atrophic gastritis. The condition is associated with malignancy.

50. (c) Hiatus hernia

This is the most common cause for a large retrocardiac soft tissue shadow and an air–fluid level within. Diagnosis may be confirmed on lateral chest projection.

Chapter 4

Genitourinary system, adrenal gland, obstetrics and gynaecology, and breast

QUESTIONS

1. A patient with urinary symptoms and raised PSA was diagnosed with carcinoma of the prostate on histopathology.

   Which of the following appearances is suggestive of carcinoma of the prostate on MRI?

   (a) Peripheral zone lesion with high signal on T1
   (b) Peripheral zone lesion with low signal on T1
   (c) Peripheral zone lesion with high signal on T2
   (d) Peripheral zone lesion with low signal on T2
   (e) Peripheral zone lesion with low signal proton density

2. A 50-year-old woman presents with intermittent pelvic pain. Ultrasound shows a cystic mass in the adnexa. This contains a hyperechoic nodule which produces marked acoustic shadowing. CT shows a fat containing lesion in the pelvis with a fluid level and a small calcified nodule.

   What is the most likely diagnosis?

   (a) Ovarian dermoid
   (b) Liposarcoma
   (c) Tubo-ovarian abscess
   (d) Endometrioma
   (e) Haemorrhagic ovarian cyst

3. A 25-year-old previously well man presents with non-specific scrotal pain. Ultrasound shows numerous bilateral hyperechoic shadows in the testes measuring 1–2 mm. There is no acoustic shadowing seen.

   The most likely diagnosis is?

   (a) Post-inflammatory changes
   (b) Haemorrhage with infarction
   (c) Testicular scarring
   (d) Testicular microlithiasis
   (e) Large-cell calcifying Sertoli cell tumour

4. A 50-year-old man of Indian origin was involved in a road traffic accident. CT scan of the abdomen shows a small non-functional shrunken kidney with extensive dystrophic calcifications.

   What is the most likely diagnosis?

   (a) Renal tuberculosis
   (b) Chronic renal failure
   (c) Lymphoma
   (d) Renal cell carcinoma
   (e) Multicystic dysplastic kidney

5. A 40-year-old mother of two presents with a right lower abdominal lump near a surgical scar and with a cyclical history of pain. Ultrasound shows a 2 cm solid hypoechoic lesion in the subcutaneous tissue. Doppler shows internal vascularity.

   The most likely diagnosis is?

   (a) Desmoid tumour
   (b) Endometriosis
   (c) Metastasis
   (d) Lymph node
   (e) Suture granuloma

6. A 31-year-old woman presents with dysfunctional uterine bleeding. Transvaginal ultrasound shows a hypoechoic vascular mass in the cervix. The mass bulges into the endocervical canal and parametrium. On MRI, there is a cervical mass lesion which returns high signal on T2 and poorly defined margins beyond the cervical stroma.

    The most likely diagnosis is?

    (a) Endometrial carcinoma
    (b) Cervical carcinoma
    (c) Focal adenomyosis
    (d) Cervical lymphoma
    (e) Prolapsed submucosal fibroid

7. A 40-year-old woman presents with nausea, vomiting and bilateral flank pain. Ultrasound of the kidneys, ureters and bladder shows loss of normal corticomedullary differentiation with lack of cortical blood flow. CT shows lack of cortical enhancement on both kidneys with enhancing medulla. Delayed images show no excretion of contrast into the collecting system.

    The most likely diagnosis is?

    (a) Medullary nephrocalcinosis
    (b) Renal cortical necrosis
    (c) Papillary necrosis
    (d) Acute pyelonephritis
    (e) Acute interstitial nephritis

8. A 35-year-old Asian woman presents with lower abdominal pain and fever. Transvaginal ultrasound shows bilateral, homogenous, extraovarian, tubular lesions containing fluid with featureless walls.

    What is the most likely diagnosis?

    (a) Cystic ovarian tumour
    (b) Chocolate cysts
    (c) Bilateral hydrosalpinx
    (d) Paraovarian cysts.
    (e) Small bowel

9. A 23-year-old woman presents with recurrent cyclical lower abdominal pain. Ultrasound shows a 4 cm heterogenous cystic mass in the pelvis related to the left ovary. On MRI, the lesion has predominantly high signal on T1, T2 and STIR sequences.

   What is the most likely diagnosis?

   (a) Metastasis
   (b) Krukenberg tumour
   (c) Ovarian dermoid
   (d) Endometrioma
   (e) Ectopic pregnancy

10. A 25-year-old woman with a history of pelvic pain undergoes a transvaginal ultrasound examination. The endometrium is 15 mm thick.

    Which phase of the menstrual cycle is the patient in?

    (a) Proliferative phase
    (b) Day 7 after menstruation
    (c) Follicular phase
    (d) Luteal phase
    (e) Day 15 of the cycle

11. A 30-year-old woman under investigation for pelvic pain has an MRI scan which shows two uterine horns with two completely separate cervices. There is a septum extending into the upper vagina. There is preservation of the endometrial and myometrial widths.

    What is the most likely diagnosis?

    (a) Septate uterus
    (b) Bicornuate uterus
    (c) Uterus didelphys
    (d) Mayer–Rokitansky–Kuster–Hauser syndrome
    (e) Arcuate uterus

12. A 65-year-old diabetic woman presents with bleeding per vagina. Ultrasound shows echogenic and irregular endometrium measuring 12 mm in thickness.

    What is the most likely diagnosis?

    (a) Submucosal fibroid
    (b) Endometrial polyp
    (c) Endometrial carcinoma
    (d) Endometrial sarcoma
    (e) Uterine sarcoma

13. A 38-year-old woman presents with painless bleeding per-vagina. MRI shows a 2 cm lesion in the cervix which is isointense on T1, hyperintense compared to cervical stroma on T2 and shows contrast enhancement.

What is the most likely diagnosis?

(a) Prolapsed submucosal fibroid
(b) Cervical fibroid
(c) Cervical carcinoma
(d) Nabothian cyst
(e) Endometrial polyp

14. A 60-year-old woman presents with progressive abdominal swelling. Ultrasound shows a large loculated cystic lesion in the lower abdomen, arising from the pelvis. Transvaginal scan shows a right side complex mass in the adnexa with cystic and solid components. The solid components show blood flow with a low-resistive index.

What is the most likely diagnosis?

(a) Ovarian dermoid
(b) Endometrioma
(c) Ovarian carcinoma
(d) Tubo-ovarian abscess
(e) Mature teratoma

15. A 36-year-old woman with history of previous miscarriage treated by evacuation of retained products of conception, presents with amenorrhea. Hysterosalpingography shows multiple, irregular, constant filling defects in the uterine cavity which cannot be obscured by contrast filling into the uterine cavity.

What is the most likely diagnosis?

(a) Adenomyosis
(b) Submucosal fibroids in uterus
(c) Polyps
(d) Asherman's syndrome
(e) Subserosal uterine fibroids

16. A 52-year-old male smoker has been recently diagnosed with bronchogenic carcinoma with cerebral metastasis. Staging CT shows a 1.5 cm nodule in the left adrenal gland. On MRI, the nodule is isointense to spleen on T2 and shows marked hypointensity on out-of-phase GRE images.

    What is the most likely diagnosis?

    (a) Adrenal metastasis
    (b) Adrenal adenoma
    (c) Adrenocortical carcinoma
    (d) Adrenocortical hyperplasia
    (e) Adrenal cyst

17. A 50-year-old male presents with history of weight loss, hypertension and headaches. Bloods show leucocytosis, eosinophilia and raised ESR. A selective renal angiogram shows bilateral, multiple small vessel aneurysms. The renal arteries are normal.

    What is the most likely diagnosis?

    (a) Rheumatoid disease
    (b) Polyarteritis nodosa
    (c) Systemic lupus erythematosus
    (d) Intravenous drug abuse
    (e) Atrial myxoma

18. An 18-year-old male presented with left ureteric colic. Intravenous urogram shows that both the kidneys are enlarged and there is elongation, displacement and deformity of the calices (spider leg appearance).

    What is the most likely diagnosis?

    (a) Lymphoma
    (b) Autosomal dominant polycystic kidney disease
    (c) End-stage renal failure
    (d) Renal vein thrombosis
    (e) Autosomal recessive polycystic kidney disease

19. A 45-year-old migrant from South Africa with history of recently treated oesophageal varices presents with haematuria. Plain radiograph of abdomen and pelvis shows curvilinear calcification in the wall of urinary bladder. There is bilateral hydroureters and hydronephrosis.

    What is the most likely diagnosis?

    (a) Bladder carcinoma
    (b) Portal hypertension
    (c) Tuberculosis of urinary bladder
    (d) Schistosomiasis
    (e) Rhabdomyosarcoma of bladder

20. A 60-year-old diabetic had a contrast--enhanced CT of the chest. He suffered mild skin eruptions and itching after the scan. The next day, he presented to the Accident & Emergency Department with abdominal pain and anuria. Plain abdominal radiograph shows smooth large kidneys with dense bilateral nephrogram and absence of contrast in the collecting system.

    What is the most likely diagnosis?

    (a) Acute tubular necrosis
    (b) Acute glomerulonephritis
    (c) Acute cortical necrosis
    (d) Papillary necrosis
    (e) Pyelonephritis

21. A 65-year-old man with known abdominal aortic aneurysm and under follow up for lymphoma, presents with backache.

    Contrast-enhanced CT shows a doughnut shaped soft tissue mass surrounding the lower part of aneurysmal abdominal aorta and the ureters are pulled medially with bilateral hydronephrosis.

    What is the most likely diagnosis?

    (a) Retroperitoneal fibrosis
    (b) Lymphoma recurrence
    (c) Aneurysm leak
    (d) Radiation injury
    (e) None of the above

22. An 80-year-old man presented with bilateral testicular lumps. Ultrasound of the testis shows small, septated, cystic lesions in the mediastinum testis, the right worse than the left. These lesions are avascular. On MRI, the lesions return low signal on T1 while they are isointense to testis on T2.

What is the most likely diagnosis?

(a) Teratoma

(b) Tubular ectasias of rete testis

(c) Epidermoid cyst

(d) Spermatocele

(e) Varicocele

23. A child was diagnosed with prune-belly syndrome.

Which of the following is most likely to be a feature associated with this condition?

(a) Polyhydramnios in mother

(b) Usually seen in women

(c) Normal bladder capacity

(d) Vesicoureteral reflux usually present

(e) Normal bladder neck

24. A 25-year-old woman presents with dysmenorrhoea. MRI of the pelvis shows that the junctional zone of the uterus measures 15 mm and returns low signal on T2 images. On T1 images, there are multiple high signal intensity foci in the junctional zone.

What is the most likely diagnosis?

(a) Normal for age

(b) Adenomyosis

(c) Endometrial carcinoma

(d) Uterine infection

(e) Gestational trophoblastic disease

25. A 42-year-old man with a history of fits presents with recurrent abdominal pain. Ultrasound shows a 4 cm heterogenous lesion in the upper pole of the right kidney, with moderate vascularity. Contrast-enhanced CT shows that the lesion predominantly contains tissue with Hounsfield units of -65 to -80. Other smaller such lesions were also seen in the left kidney.

What is the most likely diagnosis?

(a) Multifocal renal cell carcinoma
(b) Angiomyolipomas
(c) Lymphoma
(d) Metastases
(e) Multiple lipomas

26. A 60-year-old woman had a screening mammogram which shows a densely calcified lesion in the right breast. The lesion is smoothly marginated and has soft tissue density with dense coarse 'popcorn' calcification.

What is the most likely diagnosis?

(a) Breast carcinoma
(b) Ductal carcinoma in situ
(c) Fibroadenoma
(d) Fibroadenosis
(e) Fat necrosis

27. A 57-year-old hypertensive woman presents with recurrent abdominal pain. Urine shows elevated levels of vanillylmandelic acid. CT shows a large mass at the superior pole of right kidney. On MRI, the lesion is heterogenous, and appears low signal on T1 and high signal on T2 with enhancement with gadolinium.

What is the most likely diagnosis?

(a) Lymphoma
(b) Renal cell carcinoma
(c) Pheochromocytoma
(d) Retroperitoneal liposarcoma
(e) Nodal metastasis

28. A 55-year-old woman presents to her general physician with left renal colic and chronic recurrent urinary tract infections. CT of the urinary tract shows a staghorn calculus in the left kidney. Post-contrast images demonstrate multiple low-attenuation masses, almost replacing the renal parenchyma of left kidney with peripheral rim enhancement, and minimal contrast excretion from the left kidney on delayed phase images.

What is the most likely diagnosis?

(a) Hydronephrotic kidney

(b) Renal cell carcinoma

(c) Xanthogranulomatous pyelonephritis

(d) Pyonephrosis

(e) Lobar nephronia

29. A 65-year-old diabetic in shock is brought to the Accident & Emergency Department after collapse at home. He has a 6-day history of progressive scrotal swelling and pain. Ultrasound shows scrotal thickening and extensive echogenic shadows in the subcutaneous layer with posterior acoustic shadowing suggesting air.

What is the most likely diagnosis?

(a) Acute epididymo-orchitis

(b) Fournier's gangrene

(c) Hernia

(d) Normal variant

(e) Traumatic

30. A 50-year-old man with an underlying condition presents with acute abdominal pain. CT shows haemorrhage involving the left kidney.

What is the most unlikely diagnosis?

(a) Xanthogranulomatous pyelonephritis

(b) Renal cell carcinoma

(c) Multiple angiomyolipoma

(d) Polyarteritis nodosa

(e) Cortical cysts

31. A 4-year-old child was referred for a palpable abdominal mass and abdominal pain. Ultrasound shows a large heterogenous mass in the abdomen. Contrast-enhanced CT demonstrates a large heterogenous and necrotic mass arising from the right kidney, extending across the midline and displacing the aorta and inferior vena cava. There are calcifications within the lesion.

What is the most likely diagnosis?

(a) Neuroblastoma
(b) Nephroblastoma
(c) Renal cell carcinoma
(d) Oncocytoma
(e) Hepatoblastoma

32. A 45-year-old man presents with left-sided pain in abdomen. CT shows a 5 cm mass in the left adrenal gland, predominantly containing tissues with Hounsfield units of approximately -80. On MRI, the lesion high signal on T1 and low signal on STIR sequence.

What is the most likely diagnosis?

(a) Liposarcoma
(b) Adrenal myelolipoma
(c) Adrenal carcinoma
(d) Adrenal metastases
(e) Pheochromocytoma

33. A 36-year-old woman was diagnosed with complicated pregnancy on transvaginal ultrasound scan.

What is the following is unlikely to be a possible diagnosis?

(a) Deflated yolk sac
(b) Hypoechoic area behind the choriodecidua
(c) Septated fluid behind the fetal neck
(d) A very large gestational sac relative to the embryo
(e) Herniated midgut into umbilical cord at 9 weeks

34. A 37-year-old woman was diagnosed with cervical carcinoma. MRI scan demonstrates a 4 cm tumour invading the upper third of the vagina and infiltrating the left parametrium. No other organ involvement is seen.

What is the most accurate TNM staging for this tumour?

(a) T1b1
(b) T2
(c) T2b
(d) T3b
(e) T4

35. A 35-year-old obese woman with history of irregular periods and hirsutism presents for ultrasound examination. A transvaginal ultrasound demonstrates bilateral enlarged ovaries with multiple hypoechoic cysts, ringed in the periphery of the ovaries measuring 5–10 mm in size.

What is the most likely diagnosis?

(a) Endometriosis
(b) Stein–Leventhal syndrome
(c) Ovarian dermoids
(d) Tubo-ovarian abscesses
(e) Brenner tumours

36. A 36-year-old woman with primary infertility was sent for hysterosalpingography.

Which of the following is an absolute contraindication to this procedure?

(a) Previous caesarean section
(b) Reconstructive tubal surgery in last 6 months
(c) Menstruation
(d) Congenital abnormalities of the genitalia
(e) Treated pelvic infection

37. Screening mammogram of a 60-year-old woman shows a well-circumscribed soft tissue density in the left breast. No calcifications are identified. Ultrasound demonstrates a homogenous, avascular, hypoechoic lesion with well-defined margins and posterior acoustic enhancement. No internal echoes are seen.

What is the most likely diagnosis?

(a) Fibroadenoma
(b) Simple cyst
(c) Carcinoma
(d) Fibroadenosis
(e) Traumatic fat necrosis

38. A 35-year-old woman with a strong family history of breast cancer presents with a breast lump. Ultrasound shows a hypoechoic lesion with internal echoes. Gadolinium-enhanced contrast imaging demonstrates a 2 cm, non-enhancing, oval lesion in the right breast.

What is the most likely diagnosis?

(a) Fat necrosis

(b) Fibroadenoma

(c) Cyst

(d) Carcinoma

(e) Radial scar

39. A 41-year-old woman presents with a lump in her right breast. Mammography shows a 16 mm mass with smooth well-defined margins. Ultrasound shows a hypoechoic solid lesion with internal echoes.

What is the correct management for this lesion?

(a) No further management

(b) 6-month follow-up mammogram

(c) Core biopsy or FNAC

(d) 12 month follow-up mammogram

(e) Mastectomy

40. A 38-year-old woman with a history seat belt injury in a road traffic accident 1 year ago, presents with a right breast lump. Mammography shows a 'hollow' spherical abnormality measuring about 4 cm with a rim of thin curvilinear area of calcification in the right breast.

What is the most likely diagnosis?

(a) Vascular calcification

(b) Fat necrosis

(c) Secretory calcifications in ducts

(d) Milk of calcium

(e) Ductal carcinoma in situ

41. A 12-year-old pre-pubertal girl presents with vaginal bleeding.

What is the most likely diagnosis?

(a) Vaginal foreign body

(b) Endometrial hyperplasia

(c) Ovarian fibroma

(d) Sarcoma

(e) Endometrioma

42. A 37-year-old woman presents with menstrual irregularities. Ultrasound shows a right adnexal abnormality. MRI shows a 3 cm well-defined lesion in the right adnexa which returns high signal on T1.

What is the most likely diagnosis?

(a) Fibroma
(b) Brenner tumour
(c) Ovarian dermoid
(d) Pedunculated leiomyoma
(e) Fibrothecoma

43. A 20-week routine anatomy scan of a pregnant woman shows oligohydramnios. The kidneys were hyperechoic and enlarged with a renal: abdominal circumference ratio of 0.35. The urinary bladder was empty.

What is the most likely diagnosis?

(a) Autosomal recessive polycystic kidney disease
(b) Autosomal dominant polycystic kidney disease
(c) Posterior urethral valves
(d) von Hippel–Lindau disease
(e) Nephroblastomatosis

44. A 3-month-old baby presents with an abdominal lump. Ultrasound shows a large solid mass arising from the right kidney with focal hypoechoic areas. Contrast-enhanced CT shows a solid right renal mass, involving the renal sinus and multiple small areas of necrosis. There is no invasion of the renal vein or the collecting system. No metastatic deposits are seen.

What is the most likely diagnosis?

(a) Wilms' tumour
(b) Mesoblastic nephroma
(c) Nephroblastomatosis
(d) Renal metastases
(e) Lymphoma of kidney

45. A 10-year-old girl presents with urinary tract infection. Ultrasound and micturating cystourethrogram demonstrates a left-sided vesicoureteral reflux with reflux to the pelvicalyceal system without calyceal dilatation or blunting.

What is the most likely grade of the vesicoureteral reflux?

(a) Grade I
(b) Grade II
(c) Grade III
(d) Grade IV
(e) Grade V

46. A 40-year-old Caucasian man presented with a painless left testicular nodule. Ultrasound shows a well-circumscribed, encapsulated, avascular and round lesion measuring 4 cm in size in the left testis. It shows an 'onion-ring' appearance of alternating areas of hypo- and hyperechogenicity. On MRI, the lesion shows high signal on T1 and T2 sequences.

What is the most likely diagnosis?

(a) Seminoma
(b) Teratoma
(c) Torsion testis
(d) Epidermoid cyst
(e) Lymphoma of testis

47. A 35-year-old man with a facial 'port-wine stain' and history of epilepsy presents with haematuria. Contrast-enhanced CT abdomen shows vascular malformations in the kidney and spleen.

What is the most likely diagnosis?

(a) von Hippel–Lindau disease
(b) Sturge–Weber–Dimitri syndrome
(c) Neurofibromatosis type 1
(d) Neurofibromatosis type 2
(e) Tuberous sclerosis

48. Zonal anatomy of the prostate is best seen in which of the following sequences?

    (a) T1-weighted images

    (b) T2-weighted images

    (c) Proton density

    (d) STIR

    (e) T1 fat saturation

49. A 25-year-old male driver was admitted to the Accident & Emergency Department after a road traffic accident. Plain radiography shows a fractured pelvis and the patient is unable to pass urine. The registrar notes blood at the urethral meatus.

What is the appropriate management for this condition?

    (a) Foley's catheter insertion to drain urine

    (b) Retrograde urethrogram to exclude urethral injury

    (c) Micturating cystourethrogram

    (d) Cystography

    (e) Antegrade urethrography

50. A 27-year-old man was diagnosed with testicular seminoma, not invading the scrotal sac.

Which of the following lymph node groups is most likely to be involved?

    (a) Ipsilateral inguinal nodes

    (b) Para-aortic nodes

    (c) Common iliac nodes

    (d) Supraclavicular nodes

    (e) Retrocrural lymph nodes

ANSWERS

1. **(d) Peripheral zone lesion with low signal on T2**

    Prostatic carcinoma is best seen as an area of low signal intensity in the peripheral zone of prostate on T2. The normal glandular tissue returns high signal on T2 images.

2. **(a) Ovarian dermoid**

    This is a germ cell tumour which contains skin and dermal appendages. These are diagnosed by characteristic ectodermal contents of hair, teeth fat and bone. Identification of a sebum-fluid level and calcification is diagnostic.

    There is risk of malignant degeneration, torsion and rupture.

3. **(d) Testicular microlithiasis**

    This occurs when there is a defect in the phagocytic activity of Sertoli cells leaving degenerated intratubular debris behind. This condition is usually asymptomatic and ultrasound appearances are typically as described. When testicular microlithiasis is discovered, regular follow up should be performed due to risk of developing a testicular neoplasm.

4. **(a) Renal tuberculosis**

    This appearance is typical of a 'putty kidney'. This results in a non-functional, shrunken kidney and autonephrectomy. Tuberculosis can involve any part of the genitourinary tract. Renal tuberculosis is usually seen secondary to haematogenous spread from lungs. Renal tuberculosis can manifest in a number of ways including as a renal mass.

5. **(b) Endometriosis**

    Endometriosis can be found in surgical scars or needle tracts. Most cases of subcutaneous endometriosis occur in Pfannenstiel incisions. Abdominal wall endometriosis is thought to occur in up to 1% of cases. Clinically it presents as a cyclical painful lump and can arise many years after surgery.

6. **(b) Carcinoma of the cervix**

    Cervical carcinoma typically presents with bleeding and pelvic pain. MRI is the imaging of choice which shows high signal on T2 images.

7. **(b) Renal cortical necrosis**

    This is rare cause of acute renal failure with typical imaging features as given. CT is the most sensitive and specific imaging for this condition. Absent opacification of the cortex with enhancement of juxtamedullary kidney and poor contrast excretion is diagnostic for this condition.

8. **(c) Bilateral hydrosalpinx**

This is usually a result of continuous secretion of the tubal epithelium into the lumen of a fallopian tube obstructed at two sides. Ultrasound shows undulating or folded tubular structures which are extraovarian. This may be secondary to endometriosis, adhesions, infection, tubal surgery or ectopic pregnancies.

9. **(d) Endometrioma**

MRI is highly sensitive and specific in the diagnosis of endometrioma. The endometrioma returns high signal on T1 and T2 and STIR sequences due to blood products.

On ultrasound the lesion may show diffuse homogenous low-level internal echoes (haemorrhagic debris). Other features may include septations or echogenic material suggesting a clot.

10. **(d) Luteal phase**

Immediately after menstruation, the endometrium is 1–4 mm thick. In the proliferative phase the endometrium increases to 7–10 mm. It measures 8–12 mm in follicular phase and in the luteal phase it becomes echogenic throughout with a thickness of 8–16 mm.

11. **(c) Uterus didelphys**

This has complete duplication, with two vaginas, two cervices and two uterine horns.

Bicornuate uterus has a fundal cleft with the septum between the two uterine cornua comprised of myometrium. Each uterine horn has a biconvex shape with lateral convex margins. Septate uterus is the most common type of uterine anomaly with a fibrous septum dividing the uterine cavity and the endocervical canal. The fundal contour is convex or flat. Uterine arcuatus show no division of the uterine horns and have a single uterine canal with a saddle shaped fundus on hysterosalpingography.

12. **(c) Endometrial carcinoma**

Endometrial carcinoma is the fourth most common female cancer, with a peak between 55 and 65 years. In postmenopausal women endometrial thickness more than 5 mm should be investigated for endometrial carcinoma.

Sarcomas are rare in this age group.

13. **(c) Carcinoma of the cervix**

Cervical carcinoma is high signal as compared to fibrous cervical stroma on T2 and enhances with contrast.

14. **(c) Ovarian carcinoma**

Malignant ovarian tumours commonly have solid and cystic components. The solid component has neovascularisation demonstrating a characteristic waveform with a low resistive index.

15. **(d) Asherman's syndrome**

Synechiae or intrauterine adhesions were described by Asherman and are usually a result of uterine curettage or evacuation of retained products of conception. The hysterosalpingogram findings are diagnostic.

16. **(b) Adrenal adenoma**

This is the typical feature of adrenal adenoma and is seen in more than 95% adenomas. The fat/lipid in the adenoma causes a chemical shift artefact which results in significant loss of signal on out-of-phase GRE images.

17. **(b) Polyarteritis nodosa**

Appearances are virtually diagnostic of polyarteritis nodosa. The condition is characterised by focal areas of necrotising arteritis with fibrinoid necrosis and small aneurysm formation in skin, kidneys, cardiovascular system and central nervous system.

18. **(b) Autosomal dominant polycystic kidney disease**

Intravenous urogram appearances are typical due to large cysts distorting the collecting system.

Autosomal recessive polycystic kidney disease (infantile type) produces microscopic cysts and on intravenous urography, and shows an initial faint nephrogram with increasingly dense nephrogram.

19. **(d) Schistosomiasis**

Schistosomiasis is endemic in southern and east Africa and is a result of infection by *Schistosoma haematobium*. Ova are laid into the submucosa of the lower urinary tract, causing an extensive fibrosing with later calcification. Ova migrating into the portal venous system result in a fibrosing granulomatous reaction leading to portal hypertension and oesophageal varices.

20. (a) Acute tubular necrosis

This is secondary to temporary marked reduction in tubular blood flow. Contrast injection especially in diabetics with glomerulosclerosis is one of the known causes. Typically, the kidneys are enlarged due to interstitial oedema with an immediate dense and persistent nephrogram with absence of contrast from the collecting system.

21. (a) Retroperitoneal fibrosis

This is hard fibrous tissue enveloping the retroperitoneum, including the great vessels, ureters and the lymphatics. The plaque typically begins around the aortic bifurcation and extends cephalad to the renal hilum, and it rarely extends below the pelvic brim.

22. (b) Tubular ectasias of rete testis

This is usually seen in older men and is thought to be secondary to cystic dilatation of the rete testis. This is a benign condition and an important differential is teratoma. Ultrasound appearances and MRI features are characteristic. These lesions are isointense (sometimes undetectable) on T2 (unlike teratoma).

23. (d) Vesicoureteral reflux usually present

With an abnormal urinary tract, there may be failure of fetal micturition and thus oligohydramnios. This is seen exclusively in men and reflux is present in the majority of cases. The bladder neck is typically wide with a tapering dilatation of the posterior urethra.

24. (b) Adenomyosis

This is the presence of endometrial tissue within the myometrium with secondary smooth muscle hypertrophy/hyperplasia. MRI features are typically as described in the findings. Foci of high signal on T1 represent endometrial rests and/or haemorrhages.

25. (b) Angiomyolipomas

The lesions contain fat (negative Hounsfield units) and show vascularity within. With the history of fits, tuberous sclerosis should be considered as a diagnosis.

26. (c) Fibroadenoma

Fibroadenomas are benign lesions often seen in young women. With advancing age, they shrink and may degenerate. This can then calcify resulting in a typical 'popcorn' type calcification.

27. (c) Pheochromocytoma

This tumour usually arises from the adrenal medulla. Note the 10% rule: 10% are extra-adrenal, 10% malignant and 10% bilateral. MRI features are typical and with elevated urine vanillylmandelic acid levels it is diagnostic.

28. (c) Xanthogranulomatous pyelonephritis

This is a chronic suppurative infection characterised by replacement of renal parenchyma by lipid-laden macrophages. In most cases there is also a staghorn calculus with renal enlargement and a rim of cortical enhancement ('bear paw' sign).

29. (b) Fournier's gangrene

Fournier's gangrene is a progressive necrotising fasciitis in men. Thickening of the scrotal skin and air in the subcutaneous layer are diagnostic.

30. (a) Xanthogranulomatous pyelonephritis

Other options are all associated with bleeding or spontaneous haemorrhage.

31. (b) Nephroblastoma

Also called Wilms' tumour, this lesion typically presents as a large mass, crossing the midline and commonly displacing the large vessels (in contrast to neuroblastoma, where the mass encases the vessels). This is the most common neoplasm in children between 1 and 8 years of age.

32. (b) Adrenal myelolipoma

Given the negative Hounsfield units on CT and loss of signal on fat suppression, the lesion contains predominantly fat. These are benign tumours containing fat and haematopoietic tissue. Presence of fat in an adrenal lesion is highly suggestive of a myelolipoma.

33. (e) Herniated midgut into umbilical cord at 9 weeks

All other findings on ultrasound point to complicated pregnancy. Physiological herniation of bowel is seen from 8–11 weeks.

34. (c) Stage T2b

Stage 1 lesions are confined to cervix.

Stage 2a lesions involve the vagina, while T2b tumours invade the parametrium as well.

Stage 3 lesions involve the lower third of vagina and/or the lateral pelvic wall.

Stage 4 tumours are seen to invade other surrounding organs such as the bladder and rectum.

35. (b) Stein–Leventhal syndrome

Also known as polycystic ovary disease, patients may have reduced fertility, hirsutism, obesity and menstrual irregularities. The ovaries are generally enlarged with multiple small follicles measuring less than 10 mm, usually subcapsular.

36. (c) Menstruation

Ongoing bleeding at the time of examination is an absolute contraindication to hysterosalpingography. It increases the risk of infection, and risks flushing endometrial tissue into the abdomen.

Recent tubal surgery within last 6 weeks is also a contraindication for this procedure. Other contraindications include pregnancy, immediate pre- and post-menstrual phases, recent untreated pelvic infection and contrast allergy.

37. (b) Simple cyst

These sonographic features are diagnostic of a simple cyst.

38. (c) Cyst

Other lesions are known to show contrast enhancement.

39. (c) Core biopsy or FNAC

For lesions as described, the appropriate management for lesions 15–20 mm in size is core biopsy or FNAC to exclude the possibility of malignancy.

40. (b) Fat necrosis

'Egg shell' calcifications are seen in patients with fat necrosis. This can be secondary to blunt trauma or it can be post-surgical.

41. (a) Vaginal foreign body

This is a very common cause of vaginal bleeding in pre-pubertal girls. Other causes include vaginal rhabdomyosarcoma, precocious puberty, haemangioma and vascular malformation.

42. (c) Ovarian dermoid

Fibrous lesions in the adnexa are of low signal intensity on MRI. Ovarian dermoids return high signal because of their fat content, with signal drop-out on fat suppression images.

Other causes of lesions which may return high signal on T1 include endometrioma, mucinous cystic neoplasm, haemorrhagic cysts and ovarian carcinoma.

43. (a) Autosomal recessive polycystic kidney disease

This condition can be diagnosed as early as 17–18 weeks on obstetric ultrasound. The kidneys may be massively enlarged measuring up to 10–20 times normal size with an enlarged renal:abdominal circumference ratio of > 0.30. The renal parenchyma is hyperechoic and there may be oligohydramnios. There is an association with congenital hepatic fibrosis.

44. (b) Mesoblastic nephroma

This is a hamartoma and is the most common solid neoplasm in neonates. It typically involves the renal sinus and there is no invasion of the veins (differentiating it from Wilms' tumour) or the collecting system.

45. (b) Grade II

Grade I is reflux only in the ureter and not into the pelvicalyceal system.

Grade III is reflux into the pelvicalyceal system with mild dilatation of the ureter and pelvicalyceal system.

Grade IV and V are more severe dilatations and tortuosity of the ureter and pelvicalyceal system.

46. (d) Epidermoid cyst

These are the typical radiological appearances of an epidermoid cyst of testis. The 'onion-ring' appearance is secondary to alternating layers of compacted keratin and desquamated squamous cells. The water and lipid contents of the cyst result in high signal on both T1 and T2.

47. (b) Sturge–Weber–Dimitri syndrome

This is characterised by multiple vascular malformations in the face ('port-wine stain') and central nervous system (leptomeningeal venous angiomas), and orbital and visceral angiomatosis (intestine, kidneys, spleen, thyroid, pancreas and lungs).

48. (b) T2 weighted images

These demonstrate the zonal anatomy of the prostate well. The prostatic urethra serves as a reference point. The peripheral zone returns high signal compared with the central or transitional zones.

49. (b) Retrograde urethrogram to exclude urethral injury

In patients with pelvic fractures, bloody meatus and inability to void should raise the possibility of urethral injury. A retrograde urethrogram should be performed to exclude urethral injury before inserting a Foley's catheter or cystography for bladder ruptures.

50. (b) Para-aortic lymph nodes

The lymphatics from the testis accompany the veins to the retroperitoneal nodes between the bifurcation and the kidneys. The local inguinal nodes are involved only if there is invasion of the scrotal wall.

Chapter 5

Paediatrics

QUESTIONS

1. A 12-year-old boy presents with a history of recurrent abdominal pain and several episodes of malaena. He was found to have anaemia. Radionuclide imaging with ^{99m}Tc pertechnetate demonstrates focal uptake in the right lower abdomen.

   The most likely diagnosis is?

   (a) Intussusception
   (b) Appendicitis
   (c) Inflammatory bowel disease
   (d) Meckel's diverticulum
   (e) Haemangioma

2. An 8-year-old chid presents with high fever and left side chest pain. The chest radiograph demonstrates a 3 cm round lesion in left lower zone with ill-defined margins. No air bronchograms seen.

   The most likely diagnosis is?

   (a) *Mycoplasma* infection
   (b) Tuberculosis
   (c) Round pneumonia
   (d) Solitary lung metastasis
   (e) Congenital cystic adenomatoid malformation

3. A 1-year-old child recovering from flu symptoms presents with severe intermittent colicky pain, vomiting and bleeding per rectum. Ultrasound shows a 5 cm mass lesion in the mid abdomen with a 'pseudokidney' sign.

    The likely cause is?

    (a) Intussusception
    (b) Hypertrophic pyloric stenosis
    (c) Acute appendicitis
    (d) Chronic constipation
    (e) Mesenteric adenitis

4. In a child with acute intussusception, which is the most useful investigation?

    (a) Plain abdomen radiograph
    (b) Ultrasound
    (c) CT
    (d) Double contrast enema
    (e) MRI

5. A 10-year-old child presents to the Accident & Emergency Department with fits and visual impairment. On MRI of the brain, a suprasellar mass was seen which returns a hyperintense signal on T1 and T2 sequences. There is patchy enhancement with gadolinium.

    The most likely diagnosis of the suprasellar mass is?

    (a) Germinoma
    (b) Craniopharyngioma
    (c) Hypothalamic hamartoma
    (d) Pituitary microadenoma
    (e) Suprasellar arachnoid cyst

6. A 2-week-old boy was admitted with bilious vomiting. Plain radiographs show a dilated gastric gas shadow. An upper gastrointestinal contrast study shows a partial duodenal obstruction and the duodenojejunal flexure positioned in the right abdomen. An ultrasound demonstrates that the mesentery and superior mesenteric vein 'whirls' around the superior mesenteric artery in a clockwise pattern.

   The most likely cause of these finding is?

   (a) Nonrotation of gut
   (b) Incomplete rotation
   (c) Reversed rotation with midgut volvulus
   (d) Reversed rotation of midgut
   (e) Malrotation with midgut volvulus

7. A 15-year-old student presents with history of seizures. CT shows multiple cortical and sub cortical calcified lesions. Gadolinium-enhanced MRI of the head shows multiple enhancing masses in the subependymal regions. A contrast-enhanced CT of abdomen shows multiple low-density masses in the liver and a large mixed attenuation mass lesion in right kidney.

   The most likely diagnosis is?

   (a) Sturge–Weber syndrome
   (b) Tuberous sclerosis
   (c) Sarcoidosis
   (d) Klippel–Trenaunay syndrome
   (e) Neurofibromatosis type 2

8. A newborn with Down's syndrome presents with bilious vomiting. The mother had polyhydramnios during pregnancy. The radiograph of chest and abdomen demonstrated a 'double bubble' sign. No intestinal gas is seen in the rest of abdomen.

   The most likely diagnosis is?

   (a) Intestinal duplication
   (b) Choledochal cyst
   (c) Annular pancreas
   (d) Midgut volvulus
   (e) Duodenal atresia

9. A sick neonate has an anteroposterior radiograph of the chest and abdomen. It shows an umbilical catheter line traversing initially caudally and then cephalad, and the tip lies to the left of T3 vertebral body.

   The catheter is in?

   (a) Correctly placed umbilical arterial line
   (b) Correctly placed umbilical vein line
   (c) High umbilical arterial line
   (d) High umbilical vein line
   (e) Low umbilical arterial line

10. A premature baby of a diabetic mother delivered by caesarean section develops tachypnoea soon after birth. Chest radiographs show hyperinflated lungs with prominent interstitial markings and prominent horizontal fissure. These changes resolved after 3 days.

    The most likely diagnosis is?

    (a) Respiratory distress syndrome
    (b) Meconium aspiration syndrome
    (c) Transient tachypnoea of the newborn
    (d) Left heart failure
    (e) Normal lung of newborn

11. A premature baby with hypoxia was treated with mechanical positive pressure ventilation. Subsequent radiographs show worsening appearances with hyperexpansion of the left lung, mediastinal shift to the right and appearance of small bubbles radiating from the hilum.

    The most likely diagnosis is?

    (a) Pulmonary interstitial emphysema
    (b) Respiratory distress syndrome
    (c) Transient tachypnoea of newborn
    (d) Cystic fibrosis
    (e) Congenital lobar emphysema

12. A 10-year-old child presents with a lump in the scalp. The skull radiograph shows a lucent lesion with sclerotic margins.

The most likely diagnosis is?

(a) Dermoid cyst
(b) Aneurysmal bone cyst
(c) Histiocytosis X
(d) Neuroblastoma metastasis
(e) Osteosarcoma metastasis

13. A 13-year-old child presents with pain in the leg. Radiography shows a well-defined, eccentric, radiolucent lesion with a thin sclerotic border towards the medulla in the proximal tibia. No periosteal reaction seen. On MRI, the lesion returns low signal on T1 and T2.

The most likely diagnosis is?

(a) Chondromyxoid fibroma
(b) Non-ossifying fibroma
(c) Intraosseous ganglion
(d) Brodie's abscess
(e) Simple bone cyst

14. A 6-year-old girl presents with ongoing back pain. Radiograph of the spine shows a flattened sclerotic T6 vertebral body with normal adjacent discs.

What is the most likely diagnosis?

(a) Trauma
(b) Tuberculosis
(c) Langerhans cell histiocytosis
(d) Leukaemia
(e) Morquio's syndrome

15. A 14-year-old girl presents after a twisting injury with inability to weight bear on the leg. Radiographs of the ankle and leg show a type III Salter–Harris fracture on the anteroposterior view. CT of the ankle confirms the fracture. The coronal reformats show that there is partial fusion of the medial part of distal tibial epiphyseal plate.

What is the most likely diagnosis?

(a) Le Fort fracture

(b) Tillaux fracture

(c) Maisonneuve fracture

(d) Bennett fracture

(e) Pilon fracture

16. A neonate born with a history of prolonged labour has a routine cranial ultrasound which shows dilated lateral ventricles. A subsequent MRI of brain and spine is performed which show a small posterior fossa, herniated cerebellar tonsils through foramen magnum with hydrocephalus. The tectum has a beaked appearance. In the spine, there is a myelomeningocele at the lower lumbar spine.

What is the most likely diagnosis?

(a) Chiari type I malformation

(b) Chiari type II malformation

(c) Alobar holoprosencephaly

(d) Hydranencephaly

(e) Dandy–Walker malformation

17. A newborn with a history of left renal abnormalities on antenatal scans has a postnatal ultrasound which shows hypoechoic cysts of varying sizes with intervening abnormal renal parenchyma. There is no communication between the cysts.

The most likely diagnosis is?

(a) Bilateral hydronephrosis

(b) Autosomal dominant polycystic kidney disease

(c) Wilms' tumour

(d) Autosomal recessive polycystic kidney disease

(e) Multicystic dysplastic kidney

18. A 2-month-old baby presents with jaundice since birth and abdominal distension. Ultrasound shows normal gallbladder and common bile duct and small ascites. A subsequent HIDA scan shows normal immediate hepatic uptake of the tracer with persistent activity at 24 hours. No appreciable bowel activity is seen at 24 hours.

The most likely diagnosis is?

(a) Neonatal hepatitis
(b) Biliary atresia
(c) Cholecystitis
(d) Choledochal cyst
(e) Sclerosing cholangitis

19. A 14-year-old child presents with left hip pain for 6 months. Radiography shows a well-circumscribed lytic lesion in the greater trochanter with a sclerotic margin and matrix calcifications. CT confirms the findings of the radiograph. On MRI, the lesion returns low signal on T1 and high on T2, with surrounding marrow and soft tissue oedema.

The most likely diagnosis is?

(a) Giant cell tumour
(b) Chondroblastoma
(c) Epiphyseal osteomyelitis
(d) Langerhans cell histiocytosis
(e) Aneurysmal bone cyst

20. A 6-year-old boy presents with worsening dizziness and ataxia. A CT scan of the head shows a non-enhancing diffuse mass causing expansion of the pons and engulfing the basilar artery. On MRI, the lesion returns low signal on T1 and high signal on T2. Post-gadolinium T1 images show no enhancement, with the tumour involving the entire brainstem.

What is the most likely diagnosis?

(a) Juvenile pilocytic astrocytoma
(b) Diffuse brainstem glioma
(c) Medulloblastoma
(d) Lymphoma
(e) Metastasis

21. A new born child presents with failure to thrive. Cranial ultrasound shows multiple echogenic foci in a periventricular distribution. There is no hydrocephalus and no evidence of callosal agenesis. CT scan shows extensive calcifications in the subependymal region.

    The most likely diagnosis is?

    (a) Hydrocephalus
    (b) Periventricular leukomalacia
    (c) Periventricular calcifications
    (d) Germinal matrix calcifications
    (e) Congenital cytomegalovirus infection

22. A 4-year-old Caucasian child presents with loss of vision. CT of the head shows a well circumscribed suprasellar cystic mass with rim calcifications. On MRI, the pituitary gland appears normal and the lesion has a fluid-fluid level. The lesion returns high signal on T1, T2 and FLAIR sequences. There is minimal peripheral enhancement with gadolinium.

    The most likely diagnosis is?

    (a) Rathke's cleft
    (b) Epidermoid cyst
    (c) Pituitary adenoma
    (d) Craniopharyngioma
    (e) Suprasellar arachnoid cyst

23. A 14-month-old child presents with abdominal pain and vomiting. Ultrasound shows a dilated left renal pelvis and calyces. CT shows a massively dilated renal pelvis with tapering at the inferior margin. The ureters are not dilated. There is a delayed nephrogram in the left kidney with no contrast excretion in the left kidney and normal on the right. A MAG-3 scan shows a split renal function of 80% on the right and 20% on the left.

    The most likely diagnosis is?

    (a) Multicystic dysplastic kidney
    (b) Congenital megacalyces
    (c) Primary megaureter
    (d) Congenital pelvic–ureteric junction obstruction
    (e) Autosomal dominant polycystic kidney disease

24. A newborn baby born at home presents with fits. CT of the head shows a large posterior fossa with agenesis of cerebellar vermis and cystic dilatation of the fourth ventricle, filling the entire posterior fossa.

The most likely diagnosis is?

(a) Megacisterna magna
(b) Dandy–Walker malformation
(c) Large arachnoid cyst
(d) Chiari type 2 malformation
(e) Porencephaly

25. A 14-year-old child injured his forearm in a rugby tackle. The radiograph shows a distal radial shaft fracture with dislocated distal radio-ulnar joint.

What is the diagnosis?

(a) Galeazzi fracture dislocation
(b) Monteggia fracture dislocation
(c) Le Fort fracture
(d) Chopart's fracture
(e) Essex–Lopresti fracture

26. A 15-year-old girl presents to the Accident & Emergency Department with pain in the left hip region after a recent half marathon. Radiography shows a small bony fragment inferior to the anterior inferior iliac spine.

Which muscle has caused this avulsion?

(a) Sartorius
(b) Gluteus medius
(c) Rectus femoris
(d) Latissimus dorsi
(e) Iliopsoas

27. A 1-day-old neonate presents with respiratory distress. The chest radiograph shows soft tissue shadowing in the right lower zone. On day 4, CT of the chest shows multiple small cysts of varying sizes containing air with resolution of the soft tissue density.

What is the most likely diagnosis?

(a) Bronchopulmonary sequestration
(b) Congenital diaphragmatic hernia
(c) Pneumonia
(d) Congenital cystic adenomatoid malformation
(e) Bronchogenic cyst

28. A neonate presents with respiratory distress. The chest radiograph shows a hyperinflated right lung with flattened right hemidiaphragm and deviation of the mediastinum to the left.

    What is the most likely diagnosis?

    (a) Congenital lobar emphysema
    (b) Congenital cystic adenomatoid malformation
    (c) Pulmonary hypoplasia
    (d) Pneumothorax
    (e) Congenital diaphragmatic hernia

29. A 1-year-old child presents with a swollen and painful left wrist. X-ray of the wrist shows a metaphyseal corner fracture of the left distal ulna.

    What is the most likely diagnosis?

    (a) Battered child syndrome
    (b) Post traumatic
    (c) Scurvy
    (d) Rickets
    (e) Osteogenesis imperfecta

30. A newborn infant was diagnosed with bilateral hydronephrosis in utero on antenatal ultrasound. A micturating cystourethrogram shows a 'bullet' shaped dilatation of the posterior urethra and a thin urethral calibre, a thick-walled and trabeculated urinary bladder, with severe vesicoureteral reflux on the left side.

    What is the most likely diagnosis?

    (a) Bilateral pelvic–ureteric junction obstruction
    (b) Posterior urethral valves
    (c) Vesicoureteral obstruction
    (d) Primary megaureter
    (e) Megacystis–microcolon–intestinal hypoperistalsis syndrome

31. A 2-year-old child presents with abdominal swelling. CT shows a large mass pushing the right kidney and encasing the inferior vena cava and aorta. There are speckled calcifications seen in the lesion.

    What is the most likely diagnosis?

    (a) Neuroblastoma
    (b) Lymphoma
    (c) Wilms' tumour
    (d) Multicystic kidney
    (e) Mesoblastic nephroma

32. A 32-week infant born prematurely to a mother with a respiratory condition presents with diarrhoea, progressive abdominal distension and failure to thrive. Abdominal radiography shows air in the periphery of the liver and non-specific bowel distension. Ultrasound shows free fluid between the bowel loops.

What is the most likely diagnosis?

(a) Necrotising enterocolitis
(b) Intestinal volvulus
(c) Malrotation
(d) Gastroenteritis
(e) Hirschsprung's disease

33. A term neonate presents with bilious vomiting, abdominal distension and failure to pass meconium. An abdominal radiograph shows dilated loops of bowel. A contrast enema shows a micro colon with 'rabbit pellet' filling defects in the ileum.

What is the most likely diagnosis?

(a) Meconium ileus
(b) Hirschsprung's disease
(c) Imperforate anus
(d) Meconium plug syndrome
(e) Ileal atresia

34. A newborn presents with abdominal distension and vomiting. A supine radiograph of chest and abdomen shows a well-rounded area of calcification in abdomen and relative paucity of gas. On ultrasound, there is a 5 cm cyst with wall calcification and echogenic material in the cyst. There is highly echogenic material between bowel loops.

What is the most likely diagnosis?

(a) Cystic fibrosis
(b) Meconium peritonitis
(c) Normal variant
(d) Intra-abdominal teratoma
(e) Fetal gallstones

35. A 4-year-old immigrant child from Africa with growth failure presents with wrist pain. Radiograph show osteopenic bones with metaphyseal cupping and fraying of the distal radius and widening of the epiphyseal plate.

What is the most likely diagnosis?

(a) Scurvy
(b) Rickets
(c) Battered baby syndrome
(d) Osteopetrosis
(e) Juvenile rheumatoid arthritis

36. A 13-year-old obese boy of African origin presents with right hip pain. The anteroposterior radiograph of the pelvis shows an apparent widening of the right proximal femoral epiphysis and metaphyseal irregularity. A line drawn along the lateral edge of femoral neck does not pass through the proximal femoral epiphysis.

What is the most likely diagnosis?

(a) Perthes disease
(b) Irritable hip
(c) Slipped capital femoral epiphysis
(d) Juvenile rheumatoid arthritis
(e) Developmental dysplasia of hip

37. A newborn presents with severe respiratory distress. The supine radiograph shows marked shift of the heart and mediastinum from left to right. The left side of the chest contains multiple tubular radiolucencies and the abdomen is gasless.

What is the most likely diagnosis?

(a) Congenital cystic adenomatoid malformation
(b) Pulmonary hypoplasia
(c) Congenital diaphragmatic hernia
(d) Foreign body aspiration
(e) Bronchopulmonary sequestration

38. A 5-week-old infant presents with constipation. A limited-contrast enema demonstrates a narrow, saw-toothed rectum with a dilated sigmoid and descending colon. The junction lies at the rectosigmoid.

What is the most likely diagnosis?

(a) Hirschsprung's disease

(b) Small left colon syndrome

(c) Intestinal malrotation

(d) Cystic fibrosis

(e) Meconium blockage syndrome

39. A 12-year-old African child presents with chest and back pain. The chest radiograph shows cardiomegaly with loss of normal contour of the humeral heads. In the spine the vertebrae show central end plate depressions and are H-shaped.

What is the most likely diagnosis?

(a) Thalassaemia

(b) Sickle cell disease

(c) Chronic anaemia

(d) Gaucher's disease

(e) Leukaemia

40. A 12-month-old baby presents with an abdominal mass. CT shows a large hepatic mass which displaces the retroperitoneal structures but no extrahepatic invasion is seen. There is heterogeneous enhancement of the lesion with contrast.

What is the most likely diagnosis?

(a) Hepatoblastoma

(b) Hepatocellular carcinoma

(c) Hepatic adenoma

(d) Hemangioendothelioma

(e) Metastases

41. A toddler presents with urinary retention and abdominal distension. CT shows a large pelvic mass with calcifications. T2 and STIR images on MRI demonstrate a large, predominantly solid, mixed signal intensity mass in the presacral region, which extends in between the sacral segments, encasing the sacrum. The bladder and rectum are displaced anteriorly but not invaded.

What is the most likely diagnosis?

(a) Ovarian teratoma

(b) Neuroblastoma

(c) Sacrococcygeal germ cell tumour

(d) Anterior meningocele

(e) Duplication rectum

42. A 6-week-old girl presents with a persistent, non-bilious vomiting. Plain abdominal radiograph shows a distended stomach with gas with paucity of gas distally. Ultrasound shows a elongated pyloric canal measuring 17 mm, with a thickened muscularis measuring 7 mm.

What is the most likely diagnosis?

(a) Gastroesophageal reflux

(b) Pylorospasm

(c) Hypertrophic pyloric stenosis

(d) Duodenal atresia

(e) Malrotation

43. A 7-year-old caucasian boy presents with left hip pain for few months. There is no suggestion of infection. Anteroposterior and frog leg views of the left hip show a subtle increase in density of the left femoral head and a subchondral lucency seen on the frog leg view.

What is the most likely diagnosis?

(a) Sickle-cell disease

(b) Legg–Calve–Perthes disease

(c) Osteomyelitis

(d) Gaucher's disease

(e) Hypothyroidism

44. A 5-year-old boy presents with a 1-month history of pain in right leg. Radiography shows an ill-defined lucency in the proximal tibial metadiaphysis with periosteal reaction and a wide zone of transition. MRI shows a intramedullary lesion which returns intermediate signal on T1, high on STIR and has an extraosseous enhancing mass.

What is the most likely diagnosis?

(a) Ewing's sarcoma
(b) Osteomyelitis
(c) Enchondroma
(d) Fibrous dysplasia
(e) Giant cell tumour

45. A 1-month-old boy, born by forceps delivery, presents with torticollis and a lump on the right side of his neck. Ultrasound shows a 2 cm, well-defined mass in the mid-portion of the right sternocleidomastoid muscle. This is homogenous and similar in echotexture to the underlying muscle.

What is the most likely diagnosis?

(a) Fibromatosis colli
(b) Branchial cleft
(c) Cystic hygroma
(d) Lymph node
(e) Thyroglossal cyst

46. A 12-year-old boy was diagnosed with prune belly syndrome.

Which of the following statements is false?

(a) It is seen exclusively in men
(b) Bilateral undescended testis
(c) Abdominal wall deficiency
(d) Non-obstructed and dilated ureters
(e) Non-hereditary multisystem disorder

47. A 12-year-old by presents with progressive proptosis and a swollen right eye. MRI shows a diffusely infiltrating extraocular mass in the right orbit which returns intermediate signal on T1 and high signal on T2 with flow voids.

What is the most likely diagnosis?

(a) Haemangioma
(b) Rhabdomyosarcoma
(c) Metastasis
(d) Lymphoma
(e) Graves ophthalmoplegia

48. A 6-year-old boy presents with protuberant right eye and pain. Blood tests are normal. CT shows a 3 cm irregular, extraconal mass having focal area of low attenuation and patchy contrast enhancement. On MRI, the lesion is isointense to muscle on T1 and high signal on T2.

What is the most likely diagnosis?

(a) Orbital abscess
(b) Haemangioma
(c) Dermoid
(d) Rhabdomyosarcoma
(e) Epidermoid

49. Transcranial ultrasound of a preterm infant with feeding difficulties shows echogenic shadowing filling the lumen of right lateral ventricle. There is also dilatation of the lateral ventricles.

What is the most likely diagnosis?

(a) Normal choroid plexus
(b) Subependymal haemorrhage
(c) Subependymal haemorrhage with ventricular dilatation
(d) Subependymal haemorrhage without ventricular dilatation
(e) Periventricular haemorrhage

50. A 12-year-old boy presents with a slowly enlarging painless lump in the midline of his neck. The lump moves cranially on protrusion of the tongue. Ultrasound shows an anechoic 2 cm cyst in the midline.

What is the most likely diagnosis?

(a) Thyroglossal duct cyst
(b) Thyroid adenoma
(c) Thornwaldt cyst
(d) Dermoid cyst
(e) Lymph node

ANSWERS

1. **(d) Meckel's diverticulum**

   The ^{99m}Tc pertechnetate scan demonstrates ectopic gastric mucosa which bleeds giving rise to symptoms.

2. **(c) Round pneumonia**

   Typical features of round pneumonia are seen in the history. This resolves rapidly on treatment.

   Mycoplasma infections give diffuse reticulonodular shadowing or segmental consolidation. Congenital cystic adenomatoid malformation presents with dyspnoea with radiographs showing cystic/large bulla lesions in lung. Metastases usually have well-defined margins.

3. **(a) Intussusception**

   This is a common surgical emergency in children less than 1 year of age. Ultrasound can accurately diagnose and assess bowel viability.

   Hypertrophic pyloric stenosis occurs at a much younger age and does not present with bleeding per rectum. Other options are also unlikely, with the given ultrasound appearances.

4. **(b) Ultrasound**

   This is the most useful investigation as it can not only accurately diagnose intussusception but also assess bowel viability and reducibility.

5. **(b) Craniopharyngioma**

   This has a bimodal age distribution (5–10 years and 50–60 years) presenting with fits and visual symptoms. High signal on T1 and T2 are due to cholesterol crystals in the cyst and solid portions enhance.

   Germinomas are solid tumours with homogenous enhancement. They may present with visual impairment. The lesion is hypointense on T1 and slightly hyperintense on T2. Hypothalamic hamartoma is rare and arises from the tuber cinereum. Pituitary microadenoma is low signal on T1. Arachnoid cysts show cerebrospinal fluid features on MRI and do not enhance.

6. **(e) Malrotation with volvulus**

   Bilious vomiting in newborn infants is most likely to represent malrotation with midgut volvulus. The duodenojejunal flexure is on the right and CT or ultrasound demonstrates a 'whirl sign' of superior mesenteric vein and mesenteric vessels around the superior mesenteric artery.

7. **(b) Tuberous sclerosis**

This is one of the phacomatoses with the classical triad of seizures, adenoma sebaceum and mental retardation. Other findings include hamartoma of kidney (angiomyolipomas), heart (rhabdomyoma) and brain (tubers). These CNS findings are typical and tubers are seen in the subependymal region, subcortical white matter and cortex. These commonly calcify.

Sturge-Weber syndrome is characterised by multiple angiomatosis in face, eyes and leptomeninges. Sarcoidosis often affects the meninges, peripheral nerves and patients may have multiple sclerosis like symptoms. Klippel–Trenaunay syndrome presents with port-wine naevus, gigantism and varicose veins in affected limb. Neurofibromatosis type 2 is characterised by bilateral schwannomas, meningiomas and ependymomas.

8. **(e) Duodenal atresia**

The 'double bubble' sign can be seen in duodenal atresia, midgut volvulus or annular pancreas, but the absence of gas in the rest of abdomen suggests underlying duodenal atresia. Duodenal atresia is also associated with Down's syndrome and maternal hydramnios.

Annular pancreas usually presents at a later age (if symptomatic). Midgut volvulus is seen in young infants. Some gas is seen distal to duodenum. Choledochal cyst is seen in children and young adults with biliary symptoms.

9. **(c) A high umbilical arterial line**

The umbilical arterial line passes caudad into the internal and common iliac arteries and then courses cephalad in the aorta. The tip should be above the level of celiac axis (T6–T10), or below the renal arteries (L3–L5). An umbilical vein catheter courses directly cephalad on the right side. The tip should lie above the liver and not passed into a tributary vein.

10. **(c) Transient tachypnoea of newborn**

If the processes of clearing amniotic fluid from the lungs is impaired in a new born transient tachypnoea of the newborn develops. This is associated with prematurity, caesarean section and diabetic mothers. These are typical radiographic features, which resolve in 2–3 days.

11. **(a) Pulmonary interstitial emphysema**

This condition is typically associated with premature babies treated with mechanical ventilation. Most commonly, the air may leak from the parenchyma leading to pneumothorax. Air may also leak into the interstitial space and spread throughout the lymphatics and along the perivascular sheaths causing interstitial emphysema.

12. **(a) Dermoid**

    They are usually an incidental finding. They have a characteristic appearance of a central lucent area with sclerotic margins.

13. **(b) Non-ossifying fibroma or a fibrous cortical defect**

    These benign lesions typically present like this. On MRI, they appear as low signal on T1 and T2 images due to hypocellular fibrous tissue within.

    Chondromyxoid fibromas show a bulging cortex and geographical bone destruction with calcifications and septations. On MRI they are hyperintense on T2. Intraosseous ganglion is hyperintense on T2. Aneurysmal bone cysts show fluid–fluid levels and are heterogenously hyperintense on MRI.

14. **(c) Langerhans cell histiocytosis**

    This predominantly affects children and is characterised by clonal proliferation of abnormal Langerhans cells; histiocytes capable of migrating from skin to lymph nodes. This is the most likely diagnosis in a child presenting with vertebra plana with sparing of the disc spaces.

15. **(b) Tillaux fracture**

    This is a Salter–Harris type III fracture of the anterolateral distal tibial epiphysis resulting from an abduction and external rotation injury. This is seen in adolescents since the distal tibial epiphysis fuses in a medial to lateral direction and is not seen in adults where the growth plate has fused.

    Pilon fractures are comminuted fractures of the plafond. Maisonneuve fracture involves tearing of syndesmosis, posterior malleolus, capsular injury and fracture of the proximal fibula. Le Fort fracture involves the distal fibula and the anterior tibiofibular ligament

16. **(b) Chiari type II malformation**

    There is displacement of the fourth ventricle, brainstem and cerebellum into the cervical spinal canal and it is almost always associated with myelomeningocele. Other findings may include beaked tectum, fenestration of falx, hydrocephalus, colpocephaly and dysgenesis of corpus callosum.

    Chiari type I may show benign cerebellar ectopia up to 5 mm below foramen magnum. There is no hydrocephalus or meningomyelocele. Alobar holoprosencephaly shows a large single ventricle without occipital or temporal horns. There is no hemispheric development of the brain. Hydranencephaly represents liquefaction of cerebral hemispheres, which are replaced with cerebrospinal fluid, leptomeninges sac and remnants of cortex. Dandy–Walker malformation is characterised by an enlarged posterior fossa, dysgenesis of cerebellar vermis and dilatation of 3rd ventricle.

17. (e) Multicystic dysplastic kidney

The sonographic appearances of this condition are typical, showing non-communicating cysts of varying sizes separated by hyperechoic renal parenchyma (differentiating it from hydronephrosis). Autosomal dominant polycystic kidney disease is seen in adults. Autosomal recessive polycystic kidney disease shows bilateral gross renal enlargement with hyperechoic kidney involvement and usually no cysts are seen on ultrasound.

18. (b) Biliary atresia

Jaundice persisting beyond 1 month is usually due to biliary atresia of neonatal hepatitis. A choledochal cyst is seen in 5% of cases. These conditions have similar clinical and biochemical presentations.

Ultrasound will be normal in hepatitis and biliary atresia, but no bowel activity is seen with HIDA scan on delayed images in biliary atresia.

19. (b) Chondroblastoma

This is the most common neoplasm seen in the apophysis/epiphysis of skeletally immature patients. These are typical imaging features, showing a lytic lesion with sclerotic margins and calcifications in the matrix. There is surrounding marrow and soft tissue oedema. MRI overestimates the extent. The tumour is almost always benign but may become locally aggressive.

20. (b) Diffuse brainstem glioma

Brainstem gliomas form up to 15% of all paediatric CNS tumours. There is an association with neurofibromatosis type 1. They commonly present with symptoms of diplopia, weakness, unsteady gait, headache, dysarthria, nausea and vomiting. These are poorly marginated and involve more than 50% of the brainstem at the level of maximum involvement. Minimal or no contrast enhancement is seen.

21. (e) Cytomegalovirus infection

Intracranial calcifications are seen in congenital TORCH infections, tuberous sclerosis, Sturge–Weber syndrome, bacterial meningitis with ventriculitis and teratoma. Cytomegalovirus infection is the most common TORCH infection.

Periventricular and subependymal calcifications are common manifestation of cytomegalovirus infection. Calcifications in cytomegalovirus tend to be limited to the subependymal region, while in toxoplasmosis they are seen throughout the parenchyma. Calcifications are much less in herpes simplex and rubella. In tuberous sclerosis, calcifications are likely to be seen in adolescence.

22. **(d) Craniopharyngioma**

    Craniopharyngioma is the most common suprasellar tumour in paediatrics and usually cystic. Calcification is seen in 90% of the cases. These lesions contain highly proteinaceous fluid, cholesterol and blood products resulting in high signal on T1, T2 and FLAIR images.

23. **(d) Congenital pelvic–ureteric junction obstruction**

    Findings of the MAG-3 scan along with typical imaging demonstrating obstruction at the pelviureteric junction.

24. **(b) Dandy–Walker malformation**

    These are the typical features seen in Dandy–Walker malformation.

25. **(a) Galeazzi fracture dislocation**

    Characterised by fracture of the distal shaft radius and dislocation at the distal radio-ulnar joint.

26. **(c) Rectus femoris is attached to the anterior inferior iliac spine.**

27. **(d) Congenital cystic adenomatoid malformation**

    These are multicystic lesions filled with air. They communicate with the bronchial tree and are filled with air early in life. Most lesions are confined to a single lobe and are solitary.

    Sequestration does not contain air in the neonatal period and is only filled with air if infected.

28. **(a) Congenital lobar emphysema**

    Progressive overdistention of a pulmonary lobe due to obstruction. Initially, after birth the lobe may be filled with fetal lung fluid and then gradually fluid is replaced by air. The lung hyperexpands and causes mediastinal shift and flattening of the diaphragm. CT shows attenuation of pulmonary vessels as compared to the opposite side.

29. **(a) Battered child syndrome**

    The classical metaphyseal fracture is considered virtually pathognomic of battered child syndrome from indirectly applied forces during shaking.

30. (b) Posterior urethral valves

There are congenital folds of mucous membrane located in the posterior urethra. The findings on micturating cystourethrogram are characteristic with fusiform distension and elongation of posterior urethra, vesicoureteral reflux (usually to the left), diminution of urethral calibre and hypertrophy of bladder neck with trabeculations.

31. (a) Neuroblastoma

A childhood suprarenal mass with calcification, crossing the midline to encase the inferior vena cava and aorta is almost certainly a neuroblastoma.

32. (a) Necrotising enterocolitis

Ischaemic bowel disease secondary to hypoxia, perinatal stress and infections. The terminal ileum is commonly involved and the bowel loops show wall thickening and intramural air. Gas may be seen in the porto-venous system in the liver.

33. (a) Meconium ileus

Meconium ileus is almost diagnostic of cystic fibrosis and presents in neonates. Family history of CF may be present. The abnormally thick meconium obstructs the ileum and a water soluble enema may relieve the impaction. This disorder produces the smallest of microcolons because the obstructing meconium leaves the colon unused.

Meconium plug syndrome is also known as functional immaturity of the colon. It is a temporary functional obstruction which often occurs at the splenic flexure, and is a common cause of neonatal obstruction.

34. (b) Meconium peritonitis

This is a sterile chemical peritonitis, secondary to perforation of bowel resulting in prenatal leak of meconium into the peritoneal cavity. This is usually secondary to bowel obstruction and perforation in utero. Meconium peritonitis usually results in intraperitoneal calcifications, which may be focal, cystic or generalised. On plain films, the primary finding is calcifications. On ultrasound there may be cysts with echogenic walls (calcifications) containing meconium. Calcifications usually disappear over months or years.

35. (b) Rickets

This is the characteristic appearance of the growth plates of children with rickets. Features include poorly mineralised epiphyseal centres, irregular and widened epiphyseal plates, cupping and fraying of metaphysis, cortical spurs, deformities and bowing of long bones.

36. (c) Slipped capital femoral epiphysis

This is a Salter–Harris type 1 injury to the proximal femoral epiphysis and is seen during the adolescent growth spurt. More commonly seen in black males. Children with slipped capital femoral epiphysis are usually overweight and may present with hip and referred knee pain. A line drawn along the lateral margin of femoral neck (anteroposterior view) should bisect at least one-sixth of the femoral epiphysis.

37. (c) Congenital diaphragmatic hernia

This is a common surgical cause of respiratory distress. Herniation of abdominal contents occurs through a posterolateral diaphragmatic defect or persistent pleuro-peritoneal canal. The abdomen is gasless secondary to migration of bowel into chest. Intestinal malrotation and pulmonary hypoplasia is seen in almost all cases.

In neonates with congenital cystic adenomatoid malformation, the chest radiograph may show a soft tissue mass in the chest, which becomes filled with air as fluid is reabsorbed over a few hours.

38. (a) Hirschsprung's disease

This is a functional colonic obstruction characterised by an aganglionic hypertonic distal segment of bowel with associated proximal dilatation. Radiographic demonstration of the transition zone between the dilated proximal ganglionic segment bowel and the non-dilated distal aganglionic bowel is the most reliable diagnostic feature of Hirschsprung's. Other features include a corrugated or saw-tooth rectosigmoid, abnormal rectosigmoid index (normally the sigmoid should not be bigger than the rectum) and delayed evacuation of contrast medium.

39. (b) Sickle cell disease

On a chest radiograph, there may be absence of a splenic shadow secondary to progressive splenic infarction, pulmonary opacities caused by pneumonia or infarction, gallstones from haemolysis and cardiomegaly induced by a high output state secondary to anaemia. Sludging of sickled red blood cells in bones leads to infarction or avascular necrosis. Typical areas of involvement include spine and humeral head. In the spine, the H-shaped vertebra is secondary to central infarction and relative overgrowth of the remaining end-plate and is virtually pathognomonic of this condition.

40. (a) Hepatoblastoma

This is the most common primary malignant hepatic tumour in children occurring before 3 years of age. There is an association with Beckwith–Wiedemann syndrome. On CT there is a heterogeneous contrast enhancement whilst on MRI, the tumour is usually heterogeneously hyperintense on T2.

Hepatocellular carcinoma, metastases and hemangioendothelioma are very rare in this age group.

41. (c) Sacrococcygeal germ cell tumour

These are relatively rare tumours and can be benign or malignant. Calcification is seen on CT in more than half of cases, more frequently in benign lesions. Direct invasion of surrounding structures suggest malignancy.

Ovarian teratoma, neuroblastoma and gastrointestinal duplication cysts are all rare and do not (usually) extend around the sacrum. Meningoceles are cystic structures.

42. (c) Hypertrophic pyloric stenosis

Ultrasound is diagnostic of this condition, including an elongated pyloric canal (> 15 mm) and thick pyloric muscle (> 3 mm).

43. (b) Legg–Calve–Perthes disease

This is most common in caucasian boys. Initial radiographic findings show joint widening with medial and lateral displacement of the femoral head, suggesting oedema. With disease progression there is sclerosis, subchondral lucency, lateral epiphyseal extrusion and calcification lateral to the femoral head.

44. (a) Ewing's sarcoma

More than 50% of cases are seen in long bones. They are common in the metadiaphyseal region and most common in the 5- to 10-year age group. often presenting similarly to osteomyelitis. MRI is extremely useful in determining the extent of the tumour, which is low on T1, high on T2 and STIR and enhances with contrast.

45. (a) Fibromatosis colli

This presents as a mass in the sternocleidomastoid muscle 2 or more weeks after birth. A history of birth trauma may be present. This presents with a torticollis with the chin pointed away from the mass. Ultrasound is diagnostic and shows a focal of diffuse enlargement of the muscle with the mass following the course of the muscle.

46. (e) Non-hereditary multisystem disorder

Prune belly syndrome is a congenital non-hereditary multisystem disorder, almost exclusive to men (M:F = 19:1).

A triad of abdominal wall deficiency, non-obstructed dilated redundant ureters and bilateral undescended testes is seen.

47. (a) Haemangioma

These are benign tumours which can grow to cause progressive proptosis. Haemorrhage may present with acute symptoms and swelling. Flow voids, when present, are highly suggestive of a haemangioma.

48. **(d) Rhabdomyosarcoma**

This is the most common primary orbital tumour in childhood. This usually arises from the mesenchymal tissues and the lesion is usually non invasive.

49. **(c) Subependymal haemorrhage with ventricular dilatation**

The differential diagnosis is from a normal choroid plexus. However, if the blood fills the ventricle then the diagnosis is easy.

50. **(a) Thyroglossal duct cyst**

This is the most common congenital neck mass seen in children less than 10 years of age. The thyroglossal cyst typically moves on tongue protrusion. On MRI, the lesion returns low signal on T1 and high on T2.

Chapter 6

Central nervous system, and head and neck

QUESTIONS

1. A 40-year-old man attends the Accident & Emergency Department with acute onset of the most severe headache of his life. CT of the head demonstrates subarachnoid haemorrhage in the left sylvian fissure and early hydrocephalus.

   What is the most likely site of the ruptured aneurysm?

   (a) Basilar artery
   (b) Right middle cerebral artery
   (c) Left middle cerebral artery
   (d) Anterior communicating artery
   (e) Posterior cerebral artery

2. A 30-year-old man presents with a lump in the left cheek. Ultrasound examination shows an 8 mm hypoechoic and lobulated lesion with a hyperechoic centre.

   The most likely cause of the lesion is?

   (a) Parotid duct stone
   (b) Lymph node
   (c) Warthin's tumour
   (d) Pleomorphic adenoma
   (e) Abscess

3. A 50-year-old man presents with headaches. A CT of the head reveals a 3 cm extra-axial lesion in the posterior fossa adjacent to the tentorium. The lesion is isodense with brain on non-contrast CT and has small areas of calcifications within. The lesion enhances homogenously with contrast. There is no surrounding oedema in the brain parenchyma.

The most likely diagnosis of the abnormality is?

(a) Medulloblastoma
(b) Meningioma
(c) Lymphoma
(d) Glioblastoma multiforme
(e) Osteosarcoma metastasis

4. A 1-year-old child presents with precocious puberty and MRI shows a suprasellar mass attached to the mamillary bodies with a thin stalk.

The most likely cause is?

(a) Hypothalamic hamartoma
(b) Craniopharyngioma
(c) Hypothalamic glioma
(d) Kallman syndrome
(e) Pituitary adenoma

5. A 40-year-old housewife presents with severe left L4 radiculopathy. 1 year ago she had a L4/5 discectomy. A gadolinium-enhanced MRI of the lumbar spine was performed.

Post surgical fibrosis and epidural scar is diagnosed on T1-enhanced images by?

(a) An enhancing epidural tissue at L4/5 compressing on left L4 nerve root
(b) A non-enhancing epidural tissue at L4/5 compressing the left L4 nerve root
(c) An enhancing mass within the spinal canal at L4/5 compressing left L4 root
(d) A non-enhancing mass in the spinal canal at L4/5 compressing left L4 root
(e) An enhancing mass at L5/S1 compressing left L4 root

6. A 30-year-old man with a bimalar rash and learning difficulties was shown to have bilateral renal angiomyolipomas.

The most likely diagnosis is?

(a) Tuberous sclerosis
(b) Peutz–Jeghers syndrome
(c) Sturge–Weber syndrome
(d) Neurofibromatosis
(e) Fibrous dysplasia

7. A chronic alcoholic was admitted with dehydration, acute confusion and electrolyte imbalance. The patient was admitted and treated vigorously with intravenous fluids. The next day the patient went into a coma. MRI shows a round abnormality in the central area of the pons which returns low signal on T1 and high on T2.

    The most likely cause of the abnormality is?

    (a) Acute pontine infarct
    (b) Pontine haemorrhage
    (c) Wilson's disease
    (d) Glioma
    (e) Central pontine myelinolysis

8. A 37-year-old man presented with a history of intermittent headaches. Unenhanced CT scan of the head demonstrates a 1 cm, dense, round lesion in the region of the interventricular foramen. Mild hydrocephalus was also seen. On MRI, the lesion returns high signal on T1 and T2 sequences.

    The most likely diagnosis of this lesion is?

    (a) Meningioma
    (b) Ependymoma of the 3rd ventricle
    (c) Colloid cyst
    (d) Dermoid cyst
    (e) Arachnoid cyst

9. A 15-year-old boy presents with a history of epilepsy and visual loss. A CT scan shows 'tram track' gyriform cortical calcifications in the right parieto-occipital lobe. MRI shows cortical atrophy in the region of calcifications. Post-gadolinium T1 demonstrate focally enhancing leptomeninges and enlarged ipsilateral choroid plexus in the occipital horn.

    What is the most likely underlying condition?

    (a) Tuberous sclerosis
    (b) von Hippel–Lindau
    (c) Klippel–Trenaunay syndrome
    (d) Sturge–Weber syndrome
    (e) Neurofibromatosis

10. A 40-year-old man presents with gradually worsening symptoms of ataxia, nausea and vomiting. CT of the head shows a 2 cm cystic lesion in the cerebellum with an enhancing mural nodule.

What is the most likely diagnosis?

(a) Cerebellar haemangioblastoma
(b) Metastasis
(c) Cystic astrocytoma
(d) Arachnoid cyst
(e) Medulloblastoma

11. A 40-year-old teacher presents with a history of hearing loss in the left ear. Gadolinium-enhanced MRI shows a non-enhancing lesion in the left cerebellopontine angle (CPA). The lesion is isointense to CSF on T1 and T2 sequences. On FLAIR imaging, the lesion shows incomplete attenuation of fluid signal and on diffusion-weighted imaging it returns a bright signal.

The most likely diagnosis is?

(a) Arachnoid cyst in the left CPA
(b) Schwannoma in the left CPA
(c) Epidermoid cyst in the left CPA
(d) Lipoma in the left CPA
(e) Cystic meningioma in the left CPA

12. A 70-year-old man with chronic rheumatoid arthritis presents with recurrent episodes of dry eyes, mouth and bilateral parotid swellings. CT shows bilateral diffuse parotid swellings with punctate calcifications and heterogenous contrast enhancement. MRI shows diffuse cystic lesions within both parotids on STIR.

The most likely diagnosis is?

(a) Sjögren syndrome
(b) Non-Hodgkin's lymphoma of the parotid glands
(c) Warthin's tumours
(d) Metastatic disease
(e) Bilateral pleomorphic adenoma

13. A 14-year-old, short girl presents with back pain. Radiographs of the lumbar spine show reducing interpedicular distance when progressing down the lumbar spine. There is exaggerated lumbar lordosis and marked scalloping of the posterior vertebral bodies.

The most likely diagnosis is?

(a) Achondrogenesis
(b) Achondroplasia
(c) Thanatophoric dysplasia
(d) Marfan syndrome
(e) Hurley syndrome

14. A 49-year-old presents with a history of painless discharge, hearing loss and fullness in the left ear. CT shows a soft tissue mass in the middle ear with intact jugular fossa. Coronal reconstructions show erosion of the epitympanic ossicular chain with intact scutum. MRI shows that the soft tissue mass is hypointense on T1 and intermediate signal on T2 with no enhancement with gadolinium.

The most likely diagnosis is?

(a) Secondary cholesteatoma
(b) Chronic otitis media
(c) Granulation tissue
(d) Squamous cell carcinoma
(e) Acute otitis media

15. A 70-year-old male with a low score on the Glasgow coma scale is admitted to a medical assessment unit. MRI shows a large area in the left MCA distribution returning high signal on diffusion-weighted images and low signal in the corresponding area on the ADC map.

The most likely diagnosis is?

(a) Acute cerebral infarct
(b) Old cerebral infarct
(c) 14-day-old cerebral infarct
(d) 7-day-old cerebral infarct
(e) Superior sagittal sinus thrombosis

16. A 27-year-old woman presents to the Accident & Emergency Department with headaches. A CT scan of the head shows widely spaced lateral ventricles, dilatation of the trigones and occipital horns of lateral ventricles with an upward displacement of the dilated 3rd ventricle.

    The underlying abnormality in the brain is?

    (a) Midline arachnoid cyst

    (b) Agenesis of the corpus callosum

    (c) Prominent cavum septum pellucidum

    (d) Hydrocephalus

    (e) Lobar holoprosencephaly

17. A 20-year-old man presents with swelling around his left eye. A CT scan shows a high attenuation mass lesion which expands the ethmoid air cells with bony erosion. There are small punctate calcifications seen within the mass. On MRI, the mass returns low signal on T1 and T2.

    The most likely diagnosis is?

    (a) Fungal sinusitis

    (b) Chronic sinonasal polyposis

    (c) Nasopharyngeal carcinoma

    (d) Juvenile angiofibroma

    (e) Chronic sinusitis

18. A 15-year-old girl presents with symptoms of chronic sinusitis. CT of the paranasal sinuses shows a low density mass opacifying the right maxillary antrum and extending to the posterior choana. No bony destruction is seen. The left maxillary antrum also shows mucosal thickening.

    The most likely diagnosis is?

    (a) Juvenile angiofibroma

    (b) Antrochoanal polyp

    (c) Fungal sinusitis

    (d) Inverted papilloma

    (e) Intranasal glioma

19. A 25-year-old man presents with painless progressive proptosis. CT shows a soft tissue lesion with microcalcifications in the left orbit. On MRI, T1 axial and coronal images show a soft tissue mass isointense to adjacent muscles in the extraconal plane while the T2 images show the hyperintense septated lesion. The lesion avidly enhances with gadolinium.

What is the most likely diagnosis?

(a) Cavernous haemangioma

(b) Orbital pseudotumour

(c) Neurofibroma

(d) Dermoid cyst

(e) Haemangiopericytoma

20. A 50-year-old woman complains of tinnitus, headaches and hearing loss. MRI shows a heterogenous, well-defined mass in the left cerebellopontine angle producing a local mass effect. The lesion returns low signal on T1, heterogenous high signal on T2 and heterogeneously enhances with gadolinium.

The most likely diagnosis is?

(a) Schwannoma

(b) Meningioma

(c) Epidermoid

(d) Arachnoid cyst

(e) Metastasis

21. A 9-year-old boy presents with precocious puberty and headache. CT of the brain shows an enhancing mass in the pineal region with calcifications. There is moderate hydrocephalus with a dilated lateral and 3rd ventricle.

The most likely diagnosis is?

(a) Pineal germinoma

(b) Glioma

(c) Medulloblastoma

(d) Meningioma

(e) Metastases

22. A 30-year-old man presents with loss of sensation in his toes. MRI of the cervical spine shows cerebellar ectopia of 4 mm below the foramen magnum and syringomyelia of the cervical cord.

    The most likely diagnosis is?

    (a) Chiari I malformation
    (b) Chiari II malformation
    (c) Chiari III malformation
    (d) Chiari IV malformation
    (e) Dandy–Walker malformation

23. A 13-year-old child with a history of perinatal infection presents with headaches and vomiting. CT of the brain shows gross dilatation of the lateral and third ventricles with a normal 4th ventricle. No tumour masses are seen.

    The most likely diagnosis is?

    (a) Aqueduct stenosis
    (b) Klippel–Feil syndrome
    (c) Chiari I malformation
    (d) Dandy–Walker malformation
    (e) Neurofibromatosis

24. A 32-year-old man with a 3 month history of headaches presents to the Accident & Emergency Department with tonic-clonic seizures. MRI shows a 5 cm intra-axial lesion in the left frontal lobe. The lesion appears hypointense on T1 and hyperintense on T2 to brain parenchyma. No significant surrounding oedema is seen and there is no enhancement with gadolinium.

    The most likely diagnosis is?

    (a) Oligodendroglioma
    (b) Astrocytoma
    (c) Arachnoid cyst
    (d) Metastases
    (e) Lymphoma

25. A 35-year-old man presents with headache and ataxia. CT of the brain shows a 6 cm cystic lesion in the right cerebellar hemisphere with a small enhancing nodule at the margin of the cyst.

The most likely diagnosis is?

(a) Arachnoid cyst
(b) Necrotic metastasis
(c) Haemangioblastoma
(d) Juvenile pilocytic astrocytoma
(e) Cysticercosis

26. A 20-year-old immigrant from South America presents with seizure. CT of the brain shows multiple cystic lesions, with some of them showing calcification. On MRI, there are multiple fluid-containing cysts in the brain, some of which contain small nodules. There is mild surrounding oedema.

The most likely diagnosis is?

(a) Multiple brain abscesses
(b) Neurocysticercosis
(c) Tuberculomas
(d) Metastases
(e) Sarcoidosis

27. A 60-year-old man with a history of chronic alcoholism is admitted with confusion and dysarthria. MRI shows a 2 cm area of abnormality in the central pons which returns high T2 signal and low on T1. There is a rim of normal tissue around this lesion and prominence of the cerebellar folia.

What is the most likely diagnosis?

(a) Multiple sclerosis
(b) Central pontine myelinosis
(c) Infarction
(d) Neoplasm
(e) Acute disseminated encephalomyelitis

28. A 28-year-old unconscious man was admitted to the Accident & Emergency Department after a motorcycle accident. He briefly regained consciousness and then started to decline again. CT of the head shows a fracture of his right parietal bone over a lentiform extra-axial haematoma with midline shift.

What is the most likely diagnosis?

(a) Subdural haematoma
(b) Extradural haematoma
(c) Subarachnoid haemorrhage
(d) Meningioma
(e) Intraparenchymal bleed

29. A 9-year-old boy with inguinal freckling presents with visual problems and epilepsy. MRI shows homogenous enhancement of bilaterally enlarged optic nerves.

What is the most likely diagnosis?

(a) Neurofibromatosis type 1
(b) Neurofibromatosis type 2
(c) Tuberous sclerosis
(d) von Hippel–Lindau disease
(e) Sturge–Weber syndrome

30. A 40-year-old hypertensive woman presents with a neck mass. A left carotid angiogram demonstrates an intensely enhancing mass splaying the carotid bifurcation.

What is the most likely diagnosis?

(a) Metastasis
(b) Carotid body paraganglioma
(c) Lymphoma
(d) Branchial cyst
(e) Carotid dissection

31. A 18-year-old man was admitted after a road traffic accident. CT of the head shows an incidental lesion in the right cerebello-pontine angle. MRI shows a 4 cm homogenous lesion in the right cerebellopontine angle which is high signal on T2, intermediate on T1 and without restricted diffusion. No gadolinium enhancement seen.

What is the most likely diagnosis?

(a) Arachnoid cyst
(b) Acoustic neuroma
(c) Epidermoid cyst
(d) Lipoma
(e) Necrotic metastasis

32. A 42-year-old man presents with increasing headache and blurred vision. CT of the head shows a large lesion in the periphery of the left parietal lobe with extensive calcification. The lesion shows heterogenous contrast enhancement. There is a mass effect with midline shift.

What is the most likely diagnosis?

(a) Ganglioglioma
(b) Calcified arteriovenous malformation
(c) Oligodendroglioma
(d) Pilocytic astrocytoma
(e) Meningioma

33. A 21-year-old boy with neurofibromatosis type 1 complains of visual difficulties. MRI shows abnormal enlargement of the optic chiasm and intense and homogenous enhancement with gadolinium. The abnormality extends into the left optic tract.

What is the most likely diagnosis?

(a) Craniopharyngioma
(b) Lymphoma
(c) Neurosarcoidosis
(d) Chiasmal glioma
(e) Tuberculosis

34. A 75-year-old woman presents with sudden onset left homonymous superior quadrantanopia. Head CT shows a subtle hypointensity in the right medial occipital lobe. On MRI, the occipital region shows high signal on FLAIR. Diffusion-weighted images show high signal in the right medial occipital lobe consistent with reduced diffusion.

What is the most likely diagnosis?

(a) Acute occipital lobe infarct in posterior cerebral artery territory
(b) Occipital lobe tumour
(c) Haemorrhage
(d) Old occipital lobe infarct
(e) Acute occipital lobe infarct in middle cerebral artery territory

35. A 25-year-old man presents with unilateral proptosis, chemosis, reduced visual acuity and a bruit over his right orbit. Gadolinium-enhanced MRI of the orbits shows abnormal contrast enhancement of the right periorbital soft tissues and extraocular muscles. The superior ophthalmic vein is also dilated.

What is the most likely diagnosis?

(a) Carotid-cavernous fistula
(b) Graves' disease
(c) Orbital pseudotumour
(d) Optic nerve glioma
(e) Cavernous haemangioma orbit

36. A 35-year-old woman with spastic paraparesis presents with an episode of right facial paralysis. FLAIR axial images show multiple foci of hyperintense signal in the periventricular distribution, aligned at a right angle to the ventricles. Contrast-enhanced T1 images of cervical spine show multiple enhancing lesions in the cervical cord.

What is the most likely diagnosis?

(a) Diffuse axonal injury
(b) Small vessel ischemic change
(c) Vasculitis
(d) Multiple sclerosis
(e) Neurosarcoidosis

37. A 40-year-old man presents with unilateral sensorineural hearing loss. MRI shows a well-defined mass in the left cerebellopontine angle. The lesion returns high signal on T1, T2 and FLAIR sequences. On fat-saturated T1 with contrast, the lesion returns low signal and no contrast enhancement is seen.

What is the most likely diagnosis?

(a) Acoustic schwannoma with haemorrhage
(b) Lipoma
(c) Epidermoid cyst
(d) Giant aneurysm
(e) Arachnoid cyst

38. A 52-year-old man with a history of previous treated arteriovenous malformation in brain presents with bilateral sensorineural hearing loss. MRI of the brain shows that the contours of brain outlined by hypointense rim on T2 and T2* GRE images.

What is the most likely diagnosis?

(a) Central nervous system siderosis
(b) MR sequence artefacts
(c) Brain surface vessels
(d) Neurocutaneous melanosis
(e) Meningoangiomatosis

39. A 70-year-old man was admitted with left sided hemiparesis. Brain CT shows an area of low attenuation in the right lentiform nucleus.

Which of the following artery is involved?

(a) Anterior choroidal branches
(b) Posterior cerebral artery
(c) Lateral lenticulostriate branches of the middle cerebral artery
(d) Medial lenticulostriate branches of the middle cerebral artery
(e) Posterior choroidal branches

40. A 65-year-old diabetic woman presents with dysarthria and right-sided weakness. CT shows loss of grey-white matter differentiation in the left parafalcine cortex of the frontal lobe.

The arterial territory involved is?

(a) Anterior cerebral artery
(b) Middle cerebral artery
(c) Posterior cerebral artery
(d) Perforating branches of basilar artery
(e) Midbrain perforating branches

41. A 42-year-old man presents in the Accident & Emergency Department with epileptic seizure. Head CT shows asymmetrical white matter oedema in the left parietal region with a mass effect. Post-contrast study shows a large, irregular and peripheral enhancing lesion with a central area of low attenuation.

What is the most likely diagnosis?

(a) Lymphoma

(b) Metastasis

(c) Glioblastoma multiforme

(d) Toxoplasmosis

(e) Cerebral abscess

42. A 35-year-old man presents with persistent headaches. CT of the head shows a 3 cm homogenous and hyperdense mass with homogenous contrast enhancement. The lesion resolved with radiotherapy.

What is the most likely diagnosis?

(a) Glioma

(b) Metastases

(c) Lymphoma

(d) Sarcoidosis

(e) Oligodendroglioma

43. A 42-year-old Caucasian woman presents with multiple fits. CT of the head shows multiple, small enhancing lesions in the cortical and subcortical areas. On MRI, these lesions return low signal on T2 and hyperintense on post-gadolinium T1.

What is the most likely diagnosis?

(a) Tuberous sclerosis

(b) Calcifications

(c) Melanoma metastases

(d) Haemorrhagic metastases

(e) Lymphoma

44. A 52-year-old man presents with headaches. Head CT shows a 4 cm extra-axial, homogenous, hyperdense lesion which enhances avidly with contrast. There is hyperostosis in the adjacent part of frontal bone.

What is the most likely diagnosis?

(a) Meningioma

(b) Lymphoma

(c) Metastasis

(d) Glioma

(e) Oligodendroglioma

45. A 45-year-old man presents with deafness and left ear discharge. CT of the petrous and mastoids shows a soft tissue mass in the attic with erosion of the scutum. No contrast enhancement is seen.

What is the most likely diagnosis?

(a) Glomus tympanicum

(b) Pars tensa cholesteatoma

(c) Pars flaccida cholesteatoma

(d) Cholesterol granuloma

(e) Congenital cholesteatoma

46. A 52-year-old woman presents with hearing loss in the right ear. Examination reveals a non-pulsating, bluish discoloration of the ear drum. CT shows a smooth expansile mass lesion in the middle ear which bulges the tympanic membrane laterally. On MRI, the lesion returns high signal on T1 and T2 sequences.

What is the most likely diagnosis?

(a) Cholesterol granuloma

(b) Chronic otitis media

(c) Glomus jugulare

(d) Cholesteatoma

(e) Haemorrhagic otitis media

47. A 27-year-old woman with facial skin lesions presents with chronic hearing loss in the right ear. CT shows expansion of the petrous and mastoid bones with a 'ground-glass' appearance.

What is the most likely diagnosis?

(a) Osteopetrosis

(b) Fibrous dysplasia

(c) Otosclerosis

(d) Paget's disease

(e) Giant cell tumour

48. A 42-year-old woman presents with bilateral proptosis. CT of the orbits shows increased bulk of the rectus muscles and a dilated superior ophthalmic vein.

What is the most likely diagnosis?

(a) Graves' disease

(b) Orbital cellulitis with myositis

(c) Orbital pseudotumour

(d) Sarcoidosis

(e) Non-Hodgkin's lymphoma

49. A 9-year-old boy presents with chronic right facial pain. Radiography shows an opaque right maxillary antrum. A CT scan of the paranasal sinuses shows that the right maxillary antrum is filled with soft tissue with destruction of medial and posterior bony walls. No significant sinus mucosal disease is seen in the other paranasal sinuses.

What is the most likely diagnosis?

(a) Fungal infection

(b) Allergic sinusitis

(c) Rhabdomyosarcoma

(d) Antrochoanal polyp

(e) Acute sinusitis

50. A 40-year-old migrant worker of Chinese origin presents with a chronic history of nasal congestion and recent epistaxis. CT of the paranasal sinuses shows a large soft tissue mass in the post-nasal space. There is also bony destruction with erosion of the basisphenoid.

What is the most likely diagnosis?

(a) Chronic polyposis
(b) Juvenile angiofibroma
(c) Nasopharyngeal carcinoma
(d) Fungal infection
(e) Pharyngeal abscess

ANSWERS

1. **(c) Left middle cerebral artery (MCA)**

    Rupture of a left MCA aneurysm is likely to be seen as haemorrhage in the ipsilateral sylvian fissure.

2. **(b) Lymph node**

    Typical appearances of intraglandular lymph nodes are of a hypoechoic periphery with a fatty hyperechoic centre.

3. **(b) Meningioma**

    These are all typical features of a meningioma.

    Medulloblastoma is a childhood infratentorial tumour which is usually hyperdense and enhances with contrast. Lymphoma can be isodense with homogenous enhancement but usually is associated with significant peritumoral oedema and no calcifications. Glioblastoma multiforme is seen as an irregular lesion with mass effect, oedema and a heterogenous enhancement pattern. Sarcoma metastases are rare and would induce peritumoral oedema.

4. **(a) Hypothalamic hamartoma**

    Also called hamartoma of the tuber cinereum, this is seen in children less than 2 years of age. Precocious puberty is due to luteinising releasing hormone secretion.

    Craniopharyngioma presents with growth failure and visual field defects. Kallmann syndrome presents with hypogonadism in later age. Pituitary adenomas are seen in girls (9–13 years of age) and are usually prolactin or adrenocorticotropic hormone-secreting lesions.

5. **(a) An enhancing epidural tissue at L4/5 compressing on left L4 nerve root**

    Scar tissue seen after previous disc resection shows enhancement with gadolinium, while a recurrent or sequestrated disc is unlikely to..

6. **(a) Tuberous sclerosis**

    The classical triad is adenoma sebaceum, mental retardation and seizures. Patients also commonly have bilateral renal angiomyolipomas.

7. **(e) Pontine myelinolysis**

    Also known as osmotic myelinolysis. This condition is seen in people with rapidly corrected hyponatraemia with intravenous fluids. The rapid correction of sodium releases myelinotoxic compounds resulting in destruction of myelin sheaths. This is particularly common in alcoholics.

8. **(c) Colloid cyst**

Colloid cysts are seen in the region of the interventricular foramen and cause positional and intermittent obstruction, leading to hydrocephalus and headaches. The lesion is dense on CT and high signal on T1 and T2 sequences as they commonly contain large protein molecules and the paramagnetic effect of iron and copper in the cyst.

Dermoid contains fat whereas arachnoid cysts show CSF features on imaging.

Meningioma is usually low signal on T1 and high signal on T2.

9. **(d) Sturge–Weber syndrome**

This is characterised by angiomatosis in the meninges, face and eyes. Meningeal angiomas result in cortical atrophy underneath due to hypoxia. Calcifications are seen in the underlying gyri and ipsilateral choroid plexus thickening is also seen. Retinal angiomas can lead to retinal detachment.

10. **(a) Cerebellar haemangioblastoma**

These CT features are typical of this lesion.

Metastases usually have ring-like enhancement or homogenous enhancement rather than having a mural nodule. Cystic astrocytomas are usually > 5 cm, show calcifications, thick walled and have no enhancing mural nodule. An arachnoid cyst is a possibility if no enhancing nodule seen. Medulloblastoma is uncommon in adults and is usually a solid tumour with homogenous enhancement.

11. **(c) Epidermoid cyst**

This resembles CSF on non-enhanced CT. On MRI, the lesion is isointense, or slightly hyperintense to CSF. Incomplete attenuation on FLAIR and high signal on diffusion (suggesting restricted diffusion) concludes the diagnosis. Non enhancement is the rule.

12. **(a) Sjögren syndrome**

An autoimmune condition causing salivary and lacrimal gland destruction. The secondary type is commonly related to rheumatoid arthritis, presenting with recurrent dry eyes, mouth and skin and parotid swellings. CT and MRI appearances are typical as described.

Non-Hodgkin's lymphoma has bilateral solid masses in the parotids and usually has chronic systemic manifestations. Warthin's tumours are characteristically inhomogeneous and, if cystic, show mural nodules. Metastatic tumours are solid enhancing lesions and a primary would usually be apparent on further investigation. Pleomorphic adenoma is usually a unilateral, well demarcated, solid, intraparotid lesion with contrast enhancement.

13. (b) Achondroplasia

Classical spinal changes in achondroplasia are: hypoplastic vertebral bodies, posterior vertebral scalloping, short pedicles, reducing interpedicular distance down the lumbar spine and exaggerated lordosis.

14. (a) Secondary cholesteatoma

Definitive diagnosis of cholesteatoma requires CT evidence of bone erosion, either of the ossicular chain or the walls of tympanic cavity.

Pars tensa cholesteatoma typically spares the scutum and results in lateral displacement of the head of the malleus and the incus. Granulation tissue shows high signal on T2 and enhances with gadolinium. Squamous cell carcinoma also shows contrast enhancement.

15. (a) Acute cerebral infarct

In the acute stage, the CT scan may be normal. On MRI, diffusion-weighted images show bright signal and low signal on the ADC map. The signal on diffusion-weighted images increase during the first week and decreases thereafter but the signal remains hyperintense for a long time. The ADC values decline rapidly after onset of ischaemia and subsequently increase with the 'flip-flop' from dark to bright 7–10 days later.

16. (b) Agenesis of corpus callosum

This is associated with parallel, widely spaced lateral ventricles that may appear crescent shaped. There is dilatation of trigones and the occipital horn of lateral ventricles, along with a high riding 3rd ventricle.

Callosal agenesis is associated with Dandy–Walker syndrome, Chiari malformations and fetal alcohol syndrome.

17. (a) Fungal sinusitis

CT findings are typical, showing a hyperdense lesion with calcifications and bony erosion. The ethmoid sinus is most commonly involved and bony expansion with erosion is characteristic. On MRI, the lesion is low signal on T1 and T2 due to high fungal mycelial iron, magnesium and manganese from amino acid metabolism

18. (b) Antrochoanal polyp

These are seen as low attenuating masses from the maxillary antrum extending through a sinus ostium to the choana. They show non-aggressive features with peripheral enhancement. MRI shows a hypo to variable signal on T1 with hyperintense on T2 with peripheral enhancement.

Juvenile angiofibroma is seen in adolescent males with an intensely enhancing mass extending to the posterior nasopharynx. Inverted papilloma are seen in older males as a locally aggressive mass of the middle meatus extending into the maxillary sinus. Intranasal glioma usually present at birth as a very soft mass centred at the nasal dorsum.

19. (a) Cavernous haemangioma

This is the most common orbital mass in adults and is the most common vascular malformation of the orbit. CT demonstrates the location of the lesion and microcalcifications. Remodelling of the bone may be seen. MRI features are typical as given.

20. (a) Schwannoma

Vestibular schwannomas are the most common cerebellopontine angle tumours with typical imaging features as given above. These are typically benign, slow growing tumours from Schwann cells which envelop and myelinate cranial, spinal and peripheral nerves. In the skull, they most commonly arise in the cerebellopontine angle, from the vestibular portion of the 8th cranial nerve.

The main differential diagnosis is meningioma, which can also grow from the 8th cranial nerve. A schwannoma is hyperintense on T2 while a meningioma is iso-hypointense. Also, a meningioma forms an obtuse angle with the petrous bone while a schwannoma forms an acute angle. Finally, a meningioma may have a dural tail, which is absent in a schwannoma.

21. (a) Pineal germinoma (also called pinealoma)

This is the most common pineal tumour and is associated with precocious puberty in children less than 10 years old. The finding of pineal calcification before 10 years with a pineal mass enhancing with contrast is usually diagnostic. Hydrocephalus is secondary to compression of the cerebral aqueduct.

Medulloblastoma is a tumour usually in the posterior fossa, and presenting in childhood. Suprasellar meningioma does not arise from the pituitary fossa

22. (a) Chiari I malformation

Chiari I malformation is characterised by cerebellar ectopia and is frequently an isolated hindbrain abnormality without supratentorial abnormalities. 20–30% of cases are associated with syringomyelia.

23. (a) Aqueduct stenosis

There are various causes for aqueductal stenosis, however the imaging features of this condition are dilated lateral and third ventricles with a normal 4th ventricle. This is the most frequent cause of congenital hydrocephalus. Its aetiology may be classified as post-inflammatory (commonest), congenital or neoplastic (rare).

24. (b) Astrocytoma

These MRI appearances are typical of a grade II astrocytoma. Grade III are more infiltrative and show more surrounding oedema.

Oligodendrogliomas show calcifications. Arachnoid cysts show CSF density on all sequences. Metastatic lesions and lymphoma enhance with gadolinium.

25. (c) Haemangioblastoma

This is the most common posterior fossa tumour in adults after metastases. They are usually seen in the cerebellum and there is an association with von Hippel–Lindau disease. CT appearances are typically with a large hypodense cyst and an enhancing mural nodule. The cyst wall does not usually enhance. On MRI, flow voids may be seen representing draining vessels adjacent to the nodule.

Juvenile pilocytic astrocytoma is seen in young age and is not associated with feeding vessels. Metastases are usually multiple in older people.

26. (b) Neurocysticercosis

This is the most common parasitic infection of the brain and is particularly prevalent in South America, Asia and Africa. In the vesicular stage, CT and MRI show multiple, thin-walled cysts containing scolex with minimal surrounding oedema.

27. (b) Central pontine myelinosis

This is characterised by a symmetrical, non-inflammatory demyelination of the basis pontis. The underlying cause is rapidly corrected hyponatraemia. MRI appearances are characteristic with a sparing of peripheral rim of tissue. The corticospinal tracts are generally spared as well.

28. (b) Extradural haematoma

Classically an extradural haematoma is seen as a lentiform/biconvex hyperdense collection bounded by cranial sutures and associated with skull fracture. The collection may be heterogenous if active bleeding is occurring.

29. (a) Neurofibromatosis type 1

This is the most common type of neurocutaneous disorder. Common lesions encountered include café au lait spots, peripheral nerve neurofibromatosis, optic nerve glioma, iris hamartomas, axillary and inguinal freckling, bony abnormalities, pseudoarthrosis, scoliosis and duct ectasias. It is also associated with malignancies including astrocytoma, malignant nerve sheath tumours, Wilms' tumour, Rhabdomyosarcoma, leukaemia, thyroid carcinoma and pheochromocytoma.

30. (b) Carotid body paraganglioma

Carotid body tumours are the most common extracranial head and neck paragangliomas. These typically splay the internal and external carotid arteries because they arise from the tissue located at the carotid artery bifurcation. They demonstrate an intense and persistent vascular blush on imaging. The combination of intense blush with flow voids on MRI has been described as a 'salt and pepper' appearance. These tumours may be familial and multicentric and are malignant in 10% cases.

31. (a) Arachnoid cyst

An arachnoid cyst returns signal characteristics of cerebrospinal fluid. High on T2, intermediate on T1 and no restriction on diffusion-weighted images.

32. (c) Oligodendroglioma

These tumours are seen in young adults and are usually located in the peripheral cerebrum. They typically begin in the hemispheric white matter and grow towards the cortex. They are well circumscribed but non-encapsulated. Calcification is a common feature.

33. (d) Chiasmal glioma

Chiasmal glioma is associated with NF1 in 15-25% cases.

Craniopharyngioma tends to displace the chiasm rather than enlarge it. It is often cystic and may show calcification. Lymphoma is more likely to involve peripheral nerves. Tuberculosis may involve the chiasm but in the setting of basal meningitis, leptomeningeal enhancement and multiple cranial neuropathies.

34. (a) Acute occipital lobe infarct in posterior cerebral artery territory

Homonymous visual field defects result from retrochiasmal lesions, which include the optic tracts, lateral geniculate body, optic radiations and visual cortex. Unilateral posterior cerebral artery infarction results in isolated hemianopia. The superior portion of the visual field projects to the inferior occipital cortex. Thus, a partial or branch occlusion of the posterior cerebral artery may lead to an isolated superior or inferior visual field defect.

35. **(a) Carotid-cavernous fistula**

Important imaging findings include: extraocular muscle enlargement, proptosis, chemosis and dilatation of ipsilateral cavernous sinus and superior ophthalmic vein.

Graves' disease affects older ages and bilateral involvement is typical. An orbital pseudotumour is a non-specific inflammation involving any area of orbit. Orbital bruit and a dilated superior ophthalmic vein are not usually seen.

36. **(d) Multiple sclerosis**

MS typically produces multiple white matter lesions that are hyperintense on T2 and FLAIR. Characteristically, these lesions are aligned at right angles to ventricles. Contrast enhancement may be seen in active lesions.

37. **(b) Cerebellopontine angle lipoma**

The lesion has characteristics of fat on all sequences (high signal on T1 and T2 with loss of signal on fat-suppression imaging).

38. **(a) Central nervous system siderosis**

Recurrent subarachnoid bleeds cause haemosiderin deposition on the surface of the brain, brainstem and leptomeninges. This is seen as hypointense signal on T2 and T2* GRE images.

39. **(c) Lateral lenticulostriate branches of middle cerebral artery**

The basal ganglia derive their blood supply from the lenticulostriate arteries. A portion of the anterior limb of internal capsule and the head of caudate nucleus is supplied by the medial lenticulostriate arteries. The lateral lenticulostriate arteries supply the lentiform nucleus and parts of the caudate nucleus and internal capsule.

40. **(a) Anterior cerebral artery territory**

The parafalcine cortex of the frontal lobe is supplied by the branches of anterior cerebral artery.

41. **(c) Glioblastoma multiforme**

These tumours are typically inhomogeneous on CT and MRI, showing irregular areas of peripheral enhancement. Tumour necrosis is a hallmark of glioblastoma multiforme.

42. **(c) Lymphoma**

This is seen not only in immunocompromised but also immunocompetent patients. On CT, the lesion is usually hyperdense showing homogenous enhancement. Resolution with steroids and/or radiotherapy is a characteristic finding of cerebral lymphoma.

43. **(c) Melanoma metastases**

The T2 shortening effect is attributed to the paramagnetic effects of iron and copper bound to melanin.

44. **(a) Meningioma**

These tumours arise from the arachnoid 'cap' cells of the arachnoid villi.

45. **(c) Pars flaccida cholesteatoma**

This typically causes erosion of the scutum, ossicles or the lateral epitympanic wall.

Pars flaccida is a small superior portion of the tympanic membrane. Scutum erosion is common and three-quarters of cases may have erosion of the ear ossicles.

46. **(a) Cholesterol granuloma**

This is caused by recurrent haemorrhage into the middle ear cavity forming an inflammatory mass of granulation tissue. Diagnosis is made by demonstration of bony expansion on CT and high signal on T1 and T2.

47. **(b) Fibrous dysplasia**

CT appearances are typical showing increased volume of bone with 'ground-glass' appearance.

48. **(a) Graves' disease**

Graves' ophthalmopathy (thyroid eye disease) features bilateral exophthalmos with bilateral enlargement of the extraocular muscles. The condition particularly affects the inferior, medial and superior rectus muscles.

49. **(c) Rhabdomyosarcoma**

Bone destruction suggests an aggressive lesion at this site and rhabdomyosarcoma would be the most likely diagnosis in a young person.

50. **(c) Nasopharyngeal carcinoma**

The lesion is aggressive with bony destruction and is likely to be malignant. Nasopharyngeal carcinomas have a high incidence in the Chinese population. It can feature bony destruction of the basisphenoid, basiocciput or the petrous tip. There may also be cranial nerve involvement, either at their exit through the foramina or secondary to intracranial extension.

Glossary

ADC	apparent diffusion coefficient
ASVS	arterial stimulation and venous sampling
CT	computed tomography
ERCP	endoscopic retrograde cholangio-pancreatography
ESR	erythrocyte sedimentation rate
FLAIR	fluid-attenuated inversion recovery
FNAC	fine-needle aspiration cytology
GRE	gradient-recalled echo
HIDA	hepatobiliary imino-diacetic acid
HIV	human immunodeficiency virus
HRCT	high-resolution CT
MAG-3	mercaptoacetyltriglycine
MRA	magnetic resonance angiography
MRI	magnetic resonance image/imaging
PET	positron emission tomography
STIR MRI	short tau inversion recovery MRI
SUV	standard uptake value
T1 SGE	T1-weighted spoiled gradient echo
T1	T1-weighted MRI
T2	T2-weighted MRI
TPVS	transhepatic portal venous sampling
V/Q scan	ventilation–perfusion scan

Index

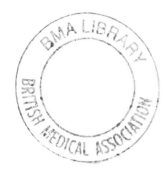